Health Promotion Theory

Second edition

Understanding Public Health Series

Series editors: Nicki Thorogood and Ros Plowman, London School of Hygiene & Tropical Medicine
(previous edition edited by Nick Black and Rosalind Raine)

Throughout the world, there is growing recognition of the importance of public health to sustainable, safe, and healthy societies. The achievements of public health in nineteenth-century Europe were for much of the twentieth century overshadowed by advances in personal care, in particular in hospital care. Now, with the dawning of a new century, there is increasing understanding of the inevitable limits of individual health care and of the need to complement such services with effective public health strategies. Major improvements in people's health will come from controlling communicable diseases, eradicating environmental hazards, improving people's diets, and enhancing the availability and quality of effective health care. To achieve this, every country needs a cadre of knowledgeable public health practitioners with social, political, and organizational skills to lead and bring about changes at international, national, and local levels.

This is one of a series of books that provides a foundation for those wishing to join in and contribute to the twenty-first-century regeneration of public health, helping to put the concerns and perspectives of public health at the heart of policy-making and service provision. While each book stands alone, together they provide a comprehensive account of the three main aims of public health: protecting the public from environmental hazards, improving the health of the public, and ensuring high-quality health services are available to all. Some of the books focus on methods, others on key topics. They have been written by staff at the London School of Hygiene & Tropical Medicine with considerable experience of teaching public health to students from low-, middle-, and high-income countries. Much of the material has been developed and tested with postgraduate students both in face-to-face teaching and through distance learning.

The books are designed for self-directed learning. Each chapter has explicit learning objectives, key terms are highlighted, and the text contains many activities to enable the reader to test their own understanding of the ideas and material covered. Written in a clear and accessible style, the series will be essential reading for students taking postgraduate courses in public health and will also be of interest to public health practitioners and policy-makers.

Titles in the series

Analytical models for decision making: Colin Sanderson and Reinhold Gruen
Conflict and health: Natasha Howard, Egbert Sondorp, and Annemarie ter Veen (eds.)
Controlling communicable disease: Norman Noah
Economic analysis for management and policy: Stephen Jan, Lilani Kumaranayake, Jenny Roberts, Kara Hanson, and
   Kate Archibald
Economic evaluation: Julia Fox-Rushby and John Cairns (eds.)
Environmental epidemiology: Paul Wilkinson (ed.)
Environmental health policy: Megan Landon and Tony Fletcher
Financial management in health services: Reinhold Gruen and Anne Howarth
Global change and health: Kelley Lee and Jeff Collin (eds.)
Health care evaluation: Sarah Smith, Don Sinclair, Rosalind Raine, and Barnaby Reeves
Health promotion practice: Maggie Davies, Wendy Macdowall, and Chris Bonell (eds.)
Health promotion theory, Second Edition: Liza Cragg, Maggie Davies, and Wendy Macdowall (eds.)
Introduction to epidemiology, Second Edition: Ilona Carneiro and Natasha Howard
Introduction to health economics, Second Edition: Lorna Guinness and Virginia Wiseman (eds.)
Issues in public health, Second Edition: Fiona Sim and Martin McKee (eds.)
Making health policy, Second Edition: Kent Buse, Nicholas Mays, and Gill Walt
Managing health services: Nick Goodwin, Reinhold Gruen, and Valerie Iles
Medical anthropology: Robert Pool and Wenzel Geissler
Principles of social research: Judith Green and John Browne (eds.)
Public health in history: Virginia Berridge, Martin Gorsky, and Alex Mold
Sexual health: a public health perspective: Kaye Wellings, Kirstin Mitchell, and Martine Collumbien (eds.)
Understanding health services: Nick Black and Reinhold Gruen

Forthcoming titles

Environment, health and sustainable development, Second Edition: Sari Kovats and Emma Hutchinson (eds.)
Principles of social research, Second Edition: Mary Alison Durand and Tracey Chantler (eds.)

Health Promotion Theory

Second edition

Edited by Liza Cragg, Maggie Davies, and
Wendy Macdowall

Open University Press

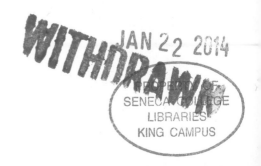

Open University Press
McGraw-Hill Education
McGraw-Hill House
Shoppenhangers Road
Maidenhead
Berkshire
England
SL6 2QL

email: enquiries@openup.co.uk
world wide web: www.openup.co.uk

and Two Penn Plaza, New York, NY 10121-2289, USA

First published 2013

A catalogue record of this book is available from the British Library

ISBN-13: 978-0-33-526320-2 (pb)
ISBN-10: 0-33-526320-8 (pb)
eISBN: 978-0-33-526321-9

Library of Congress Cataloging-in-Publication Data
CIP data applied for

Typesetting and e-book compilations by
RefineCatch Limited, Bungay, Suffolk

Fictitious names of companies, products, people, characters and/or data that may be used herein (in case studies or in examples) are not intended to represent any real individual, company, product or event.

Praise for this book

"Health Promotion Theory *authoritatively guides the reader through the history of health promotion, its underlying politics, values and theoretical perspectives. New information is introduced in easily digestible chunks, before being reinforced with simple, effective learning activities. The book will make an excellent contribution to foundational learning and teaching in* Health Promotion."

"*A readable and engaging overview of health promotion theory and practice from a public health perspective. This book offers an excellent starting point for those wanting to develop their appreciation of what health promotion entails.*"

Contents

List of figures, tables, and boxes

Figures

Tables

Boxes

List of authors

Franklin Apfel is Managing Director of World Health Communication Associates

Virginia Berridge is Professor of History and Director of the Centre for History in Public Health at the London School of Hygiene & Tropical Medicine

Sara Cooper is a PhD candidate at the London School of Hygiene & Tropical Medicine

Liza Cragg is a freelance consultant specializing in international health

Maggie Davies is Executive Director of Health Action Partnership International

Nick Fahy is Director of Nick Fahy Consulting Ltd.

Adam Fletcher is a senior lecturer in Social Science and Health at the Centre for the Development and Evaluation of Complex Interventions for Public Health Improvement, Cardiff University School of Social Sciences

Ford Hickson is a lecturer at the London School of Hygiene & Tropical Medicine

Anis Kazi is a public health researcher

Wendy Macdowall is a lecturer in Health Promotion at the London School of Hygiene & Tropical Medicine

Alex Mold is a lecturer at the Centre for History in Public Health at the London School of Hygiene & Tropical Medicine

Antony Morgan is a Visiting Professor, Glasgow Caledonian University

Don Nutbeam is Professor of Public Health and Vice Chancellor, University of Southampton

Mark Petticrew is Professor of Public Health Evaluation at the London School of Hygiene & Tropical Medicine

Morten Skovdal is a research fellow at the Department of Health Promotion and Development, University of Bergen

Nicki Thorogood is a senior lecturer in Sociology at the London School of Hygiene & Tropical Medicine

Acknowledgements

This book is based on the distance learning and in-house modules on Health Promotion Theory at the London School of Hygiene & Tropical Medicine, which have evolved over many years under the influence of Melvyn Hillsdon, Dalya Marks, Christopher Bonell, and many others. The editors are grateful for input from Rosalind Plowman, Nicki Thorogood, Adam Fletcher, and Andrew Rodgers. We would also like to thank the students and teaching staff who provided useful feedback on the first edition of this book, which has been used to inform the development of this second edition.

We would like to express our grateful thanks to the following copyright holders for granting permission to reproduce material in this book.

Overview of the book

Introduction

Since the early nineteenth century, the health of the public has improved dramatically in many parts of the world, though in some countries the rate of change has been more significant than in others. These improvements in health are a consequence of three main developments:

- improved levels of health care;
- the implementation of public policies and legislation designed to improve social and environmental conditions; and
- the formation of health promotion strategies, including prevention services (for example, services to increase awareness of the health risks of smoking).

This book focuses on the theoretical basis of the third of these three main contributors: health promotion.

Focusing as it does on theory, this book is of relevance to low-, middle-, and high-income countries. However, given that much of the literature has been produced in high-income countries, there is inevitably an apparent emphasis on those regions of the world. Its important to recognize that most of the ideas and concepts, while originating in high-income countries, are equally relevant when considering health promotion initiatives in low- and middle-income countries. Although actions will differ according to identified need and cultural specificity in countries, this book provides the underpinning theory on which a range of interventions can be built.

Why study health promotion theory?

Health promotion has been defined as the process of enabling people to increase control over, and to improve, their health (WHO, 1986). Given the emphasis this implies on *action*, it may not immediately be obvious why public health practitioners and students of public health should spend time learning about the *theory* of health promotion. However, as this book makes clear, health promotion is far from straightforward. Unless public health practitioners understand the theory underpinning health promotion and use it to inform their practice, there is a real risk, at best, of establishing ineffective interventions and, at worst, of antagonizing and even harming the very people they are seeking to help.

This book will guide you through the origins and development of health promotion and enable you to explore how this development has been influenced by philosophical, ethical, and political debates. It will explain a range of theories, frameworks, and methodologies that have been developed to help understand public health problems and develop effective health promotion responses to these. Throughout the book, the focus remains firmly on assisting you in applying the ideas and concepts described to practical implementation of health promotion activities in your own context.

Structure of the book

This book is structured in two Sections. Section 1, which is made up of four chapters, explores the history of health promotion and the theoretical concepts that underpin it. Section 2, which consists of six chapters, looks at how to use theory in health promotion practice.

Each chapter follows the same format. A brief overview tells you about the contents, followed by learning objectives and the key terms you will encounter. There are several activities in each chapter, which are designed to provoke or challenge certain concepts, or to test knowledge and understanding. Each activity is followed by feedback to enable you to check on your own understanding. If things are not clear, then you are encouraged to go back and re-read the material.

Section 1: History and concepts of health promotion

Chapter 1 explores the history of health promotion within the context of the development of public health from the nineteenth century to the present. It explains that 'health promotion' as a specific concept came into use in the 1980s, but to understand its meaning and significance we need to see health promotion in the context of the broader history of public health. Chapter 2 introduces social constructionism as a particular conceptual framework and explains how it might be used to make explicit the concepts and assumptions that underpin 'health promotion'. This enables us to look critically at the whole health promotion endeavour and to consider what role it plays and what consequences it might have in society more generally.

Chapter 3 discusses what drives health promotion. In particular, it explores how evidence is generated and used in health promotion. Chapter 4 explores political and ethical issues raised by health promotion, including the relationship between individuals and society, who has the right to decide, and the basis on which health promotion is justified. It goes on to discuss different theoretical approaches for resolving these issues.

Section 2: Using theory to inform health promotion practice

Chapter 5 provides an overview of the use of theory to guide health promotion and demonstrates how theories can greatly enhance the effectiveness and sustainability of health promotion programmes. It also explores how theory can be directed towards achieving change at the individual level. Chapter 6 explores the importance of the community in translating health promotion messages into action. It describes how theory can help us understand the best ways to engage with local communities to provide more health-enabling social environments and to enable the health-promoting role of the community.

Chapter 7 discusses the range of factors that have an impact on the ability of individuals, communities, and societies to develop and maintain good health and well-being. It explores conceptual models for understanding these determinants of health and explains how such models are used in practice. Chapter 8 highlights the nature and extent of health inequalities. It introduces a range of theoretical perspectives that have been proposed to explain these inequalities and discusses how these can inform health promotion approaches and methods. Chapter 9 gives an overview of the Rose hypothesis, a theory developed to make health promotion more effective by addressing the distribution of risk in the population. It then explores the benefits and limitations of whole population and targeted approaches.

Finally, Chapter 10 discusses the importance of health communication and describes how it has moved from the margins to the centre of health promotion practice. It explores the theoretical and contextual factors that have driven this change and introduces a selection of current health communication practices, approaches, and opportunities.

Reference

World Health Organization (WHO) (1986) *The Ottawa Charter for Health Promotion*. Available at: http://www.who.int/healthpromotion/conferences/previous/ottawa/en/ [accessed 18 October 2012].

SECTION 1

History and concepts of health promotion

The history of health promotion

Alex Mold and Virginia Berridge

Overview

In this chapter, you will explore the history of health promotion within the context of the development of public health from the nineteenth century to the present. You will learn that 'health promotion' as a specific concept came in to use in the 1980s, but to understand its meaning and significance you need to see health promotion in the light of the broader history of public health and changes in its definition over time. Three crucial phases are identified. The first phase took place during the nineteenth century, a period when promoting good health was part of the broader development of public health measures in the West, such as the improvement of sanitation. The second phase occurred in the early to mid twentieth century, a time when the focus of public health shifted away from the environment as a cause of ill health and began instead to focus on families and individuals. The third phase encompasses the late twentieth century and beyond. This is the period of the 'new public health', characterized by its focus on prevention, risk and the environment, and of health promotion as a national and international movement. Finally, you will assess some of the critiques levelled at health promotion, and you will see that these can be related to the past just as much as the present.

Learning objectives

After reading this chapter, you will be able to:

- describe the historical roots of the current concept of health promotion
- place changing definitions of public health and health promotion in social, economic, and political context
- evaluate political and scientific critiques of health promotion

Key terms

Eugenics: The science of human heredity, informed by evolutionary theory. In the early twentieth century, eugenics was concerned with racial improvement and the prevention of degeneration.

Health promotion: The process of enabling people to increase control over, and to improve, their health (WHO, 1986).

New public health: Form of public health that developed from the 1970s onwards. Emphasized risk, prevention, and individual behaviour as a cause of disease.

Primary health care: Health services and care delivered at the local level often through community health workers, which has been particularly important in the global south from the 1970s onwards.

Social medicine: Form of public health developed in the inter-war years. Concerned with the effect of social conditions on health and mortality.

Introduction

'Health promotion' is a relatively new term, but it is an old concept. The phrase 'health promotion' was first used at national and international policy levels during the 1980s (Berridge 2010), but promoting good health as an idea has been around for as long as there have been attempts to improve the public's health. One of the earliest public health texts, Hippocrates' *On Airs, Waters and Places* (written around 400 B.C.) was intended as a guide for settlers going to new environments to help prevent them from getting sick (Porter, 1999: 15–16). To understand health promotion, and its place within contemporary public health, you need to know where it came from and how it developed. Health promotion and public health are not static concepts, and after reading this chapter you will be able to explain how and why these have changed over time. By learning about the history of public health and health promotion, you will be better equipped to deal with the problems that health promotion faces today and also be able to envision where it might go next.

Activity 1.1

This activity encourages you to reflect on how the meanings of both public health and health promotion have changed over time. Your task is to read the three quotations below and decide when you think these statements were made. Each extract is taken from a key document from the history of health promotion since the nineteenth century. One is from 1843, one is from 1943, and one is from 1976. Which is which? What are your reasons for dating the extracts in this way?

Extract 1: 'we need to interest individuals, communities and society as a whole in the idea that prevention is better than cure'.

Extract 2: 'The primary and most important measures, and at the same time the most practicable … are drainage, the removal of refuse from habitations, streets and roads, and the improvement of supplies of water.'

Extract 3: 'There is no sharp division between individual and social medicine. Health education and periodic health examination will some day supplement the remedial activities of the general practitioner.'

Feedback

Extract 1 is from 1976, Extract 2 is from 1843, and Extract 3 is from 1943.

You might have decided that the first extract was the most recent one because of its emphasis on the idea that prevention is better than cure. Indeed, this extract is taken from the UK Department of Health's (1976) report, *Prevention and Health: Everybody's Business*, which was indicative of the greater emphasis being placed on preventive measures as part of the new public health, the third phase in the evolution of health promotion discussed in this chapter.

You might have thought that the second extract was from 1842 because of its foregrounding of environmental factors. The extract, which comes from Edwin Chadwick's (1843) *Report on the Sanitary Condition of the Labouring Population of Great Britain*, is typical of nineteenth-century public health that focused on sanitation and the environment as both the cause and the solution to public health problems. But, as you will see, the environment made a re-appearance (albeit in a different way) in recent formulations of health promotion.

By the process of elimination, the third extract must be from 1943 (Ryle, 1943), but the clue to the date here is the use of the term 'social medicine', a concept that was integral to public health in the middle of the twentieth century. The emergence of social medicine was one aspect of the second phase in the development of public health discussed in this chapter. Each extract thus typifies one of the three phases that you are going to explore in more detail.

Phase 1: The nineteenth century

Environment and sanitation

Over the course of the nineteenth century, the populations of Britain and other Western nations grew rapidly. The population of Europe expanded from 123 million in 1800 to 230 million by 1890 (de Vries, 1984: 36). Moreover, this population growth was accompanied by industrialization and urbanization. The number of people living in towns and cities expanded as they left the countryside to find jobs in the new factories. This process was most pronounced in Britain, the heart of the Industrial Revolution. Small towns like Birmingham in the West Midlands became large cities: the population of Birmingham increased more than seven-fold between 1800 and 1900, from 74,000 to over 522,000. Major cities like London grew even larger: in 1831 the population of London was around 1.6 million, but by 1871 it had doubled to 3.2 million (UK Census).

Living and working conditions in these rapidly expanding cities were extremely poor, as key facilities, such as housing and sanitation, did not keep pace with the growth in population. For example, in 1840 the River Aire in Leeds was described as 'a reservoir of poison carefully kept for the purpose of breeding a pestilence in the town' and was composed of 'refuse from water closets, cesspools, privies, common drains, dung-hill drainings, infirmary refuse, wastes from slaughter houses, chemical soap, gas, dye houses and manufacturers, coloured by blue and black dye, pig manure, old urine wash, there were dead animals, vegetable substances and occasionally a decomposed human body' (quoted in Wohl, 1983: 235). In these conditions, infectious diseases thrived. Throughout the nineteenth century, there were a series of epidemics of diseases such as cholera and typhoid; around 53,000 people died in England and Wales in the 1848 cholera outbreak alone (Snow, 2002).

The environment, perhaps unsurprisingly, was seen as a cause of disease. However, in the early part of the nineteenth century it was widely believed that disease was caused by bad smells and noxious gases – what was called 'miasma'. Such beliefs were undermined eventually by the investigations of men like John Snow, who in 1854 deduced that cholera was a waterborne disease. Although it took some time for Snow's findings to be accepted, by the second half of the nineteenth century sanitarian reform was well underway (Hamlin, 1998). Measures such as the removal of sewage and other refuse and the provision of clean water were paid for by the more affluent city dwellers and by municipal governments (Melosi, 2000).

Social control?

Such actions were not, however, rooted solely in altruism. Although the middle and upper classes that lived in urban areas could, of course, also be exposed to infectious diseases, they were driven to take measures to improve public health for socio-political reasons as well. Epidemic disease posed a threat to the nation's health, but also to its political, social, and economic well-being. Sick individuals were less able to work and so generate wealth, or to perform military duties and protect the nation and its empire. Political leaders therefore began to develop a series of public health policies that were intended to secure the health of the working population. Measures such as compulsory vaccination against smallpox were introduced, despite considerable popular and scientific opposition (Hennock, 1998; Durbach, 2005). The notification of incidences of infectious diseases was also made obligatory, as was treatment for some conditions, most notably venereal disease (what we would now call sexually transmitted infections) among women suspected of being prostitutes, but not their male clients. This double standard, and the fact that public health measures were often targeted at specific sections of society, has led some historians to see public health in this period as a form of social control (Donajgrodzki, 1977). Other historians, such as Christopher Hamlin, have argued that nineteenth-century public health focused on technical solutions rather than addressing the causal factors underlying public health problems, such as poverty (Hamlin, 1998).

Activity 1.2

In this activity, you will consider historical approaches to public health through a case study on sanitation and public health in the nineteenth century. Read the extracts below, and then answer the questions that follow.

'consider the kind of public health that arose in Britain, one pre-occupied with water and wastes. It is difficult to acknowledge a need to explain this for it remains a central and uncontroversial part of public health. The water and sewage technologies the sanitarians developed quickly became one of the most widely diffused technological complexes in human history … That we no longer see this achievement as revolutionary shows only how well the revolutionaries "black boxed" it. A world in which modern sanitation would have been rejected is unthinkable – the overflowing privy transcends ideology, calling only for a minimally competent engineer.' (p. 7)

'the early Victorians invented one public health among many. Their sanitary movement was not a systematic campaign to eliminate excess mortality. Its concern was with *some* aspects [original italics] of the health of some [original italics] people: working-class men of working age. Women, infants, children and the aged were largely ignored.' (p. 12)

'Chadwick and company rejected work, wages, and food to focus on water and filth, arguably the greatest "technical fix" in history.' (p. 13)

(Extracts taken from Christopher Hamlin (1998) Public Health and Social Justice in the Age of Chadwick, Britain 1800–1854. Cambridge, Cambridge University Press.)

1 What argument is Hamlin making about sanitation in nineteenth-century Britain?
2 What, according to Hamlin, would an alternative vision of public health have looked like at this time?

Feedback

Hamlin is arguing that sanitation was central to nineteenth-century ideas about public health in Britain. He states that the technologies developed – such as the removal of sewage and the provision of clean water – were one of the most successful innovations of all time. So successful, in fact, that we can no longer see how revolutionary these were, or acknowledge that it is necessary to explain how and why these measures came in to being.

Hamlin suggests that the Victorian fixation on sanitation meant that other factors also crucial to public health were ignored. An alternative vision of public health in this period would have concentrated on reducing mortality for the whole population, not just among men of working age. This, Hamlin suggests, could have been achieved by focusing on improvements such as higher wages and better nutrition. In other words, social conditions were as important as the environment as a cause of ill health. We will return to this argument later when we consider some of the challenges faced by health promotion in the contemporary period.

The bacteriological revolution

Towards the end of the nineteenth century, environmental understandings of public health were pushed in a new, more specific direction. During the 1880s, the work of Louis Pasteur in France and Robert Koch in Germany demonstrated that micro-organisms (bacteria) caused many forms of infectious disease. Their discoveries resulted in a significant growth in laboratory and scientific medicine, and led eventually to the development of effective drug treatments, in the form of antibiotics, although this was not until the 1940s. Some historians dispute the extent to which this constituted a 'bacteriological revolution', but these developments did lead to a 'narrower concept of dirt' and to a more specific understanding of the kinds of material that cause illness (Worboys, 2000). It has been suggested that the bacteriological revolution resulted in a stronger focus on the individual and the disease rather than on cleansing the environment. However, other historians have argued against this, asserting that this was actually a new form of environmentalism that stressed the individual's place in the environment (Porter, 1999). Indeed, by the early twentieth century, attention was shifting towards a focus on a different kind of hygiene, not in the sense of drains and waste, but on what was called 'social hygiene'.

Phase 2: 1900–1970

Social hygiene

Social hygiene was concerned with the social influences on individual and public health, and aimed to encourage a focus on preventive medicine. Underpinning this social focus, however, was a strong reliance on biological determinism. Proponents of social hygiene believed that the health and behaviour of individuals was determined by inherited traits and characteristics. Social hygienists thought that such conditions as alcoholism, and many other kinds of physical and mental illnesses, were passed on through the generations. The concept of health was tied strongly to ideas about national efficiency in this period. There was little sign of what we would now see as a notion of positive health, as health being more than the absence of disease. Fears about national efficiency coalesced around the concept of 'degeneration': the belief that bad breeding was weakening the 'race'. The Boer War (1899–1902) brought these issues into focus in Britain, as large numbers of army recruits were found to be unfit to fight; and the supposedly mighty British Army had trouble defeating a few Boer farmers (Jones, 1986).

To overcome such weaknesses, eugenic approaches were adopted. Eugenics was the science of improving the health of the population through controlled breeding (Bashford and Levine, 2010). Eugenic ideas led to the development of what we would now see as reprehensible policies, such as the forced sterilization of those believed to be 'unfit' to have children, including alcoholics and individuals with learning difficulties and mental health problems. At the same time, there was also a strong emphasis placed on improving maternity services and reducing infant mortality and morbidity. Attempts were made to encourage mothers to breastfeed, to produce better meals, and to reach higher standards of hygiene in the home (Apple, 1987). Maternal ignorance and poor personal hygiene were blamed frequently for infant deaths, yet the highest infant mortality was often concentrated in the poorest areas (Dyhouse, 1978).

The focus on motherhood and child health resulted in such developments as the introduction of health visitors, women who would enter homes and advise mothers on matters such as feeding, hygiene, and good parenting. Health visitors could be seen as intruding into the lives of the working class, another form of social control whereby the elite sought to regulate the behaviour of those lower down the social order. Some historians, however, have shown that by the inter-war period health visitors became more accepted and were offering support and advice to women in need (Davies, 1988).

Activity 1.3

This activity looks at early twentieth-century approaches to improving maternal and child health. Examine the image in Figure 1.1, which is a reproduction of a leaflet produced by the East and West Molesey Infant Welfare Centre in Surrey, England circa 1930, and then answer the following questions:

1 Who do you think the leaflet was targeted at?
2 What effect do you think it might have had on its audience?

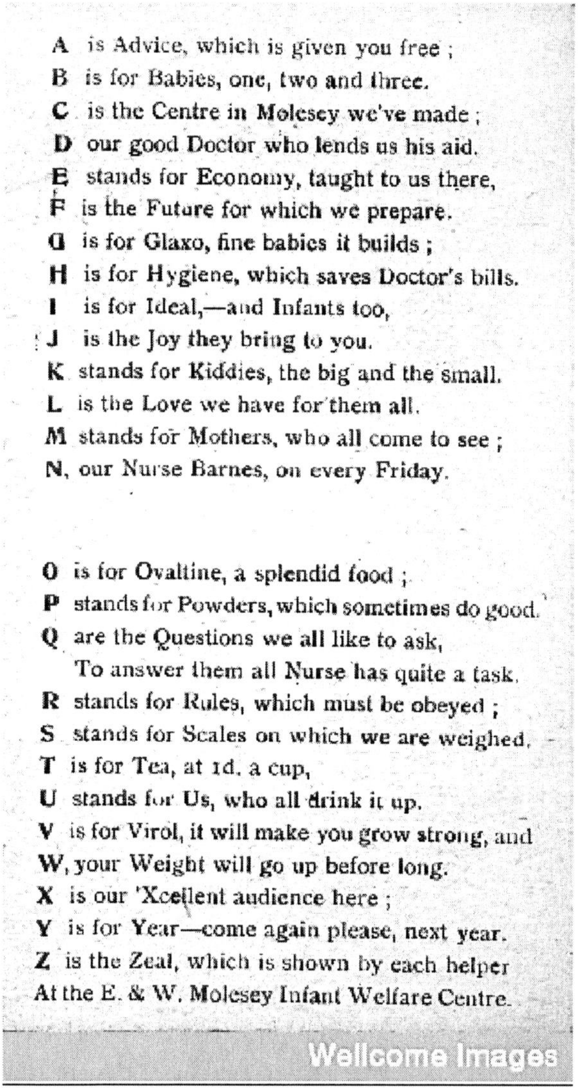

A   is Advice, which is given you free ;
B   is for Babies, one, two and three.
C   is the Centre in Molesey we've made ;
D   our good Doctor who lends us his aid.
E   stands for Economy, taught to us there,
F   is the Future for which we prepare.
G   is for Glaxo, fine babies it builds ;
H   is for Hygiene, which saves Doctor's bills.
I   is for Ideal,—and Infants too,
J   is the Joy they bring to you.
K   stands for Kiddies, the big and the small.
L   is the Love we have for them all.
M   stands for Mothers, who all come to see ;
N, our Nurse Barnes, on every Friday.

O   is for Ovaltine, a splendid food ;
P   stands for Powders, which sometimes do good.
Q   are the Questions we all like to ask,
      To answer them all Nurse has quite a task.
R   stands for Rules, which must be obeyed ;
S   stands for Scales on which we are weighed.
T   is for Tea, at 1d. a cup,
U   stands for Us, who all drink it up.
V   is for Virol, it will make you grow strong, and
W, your Weight will go up before long.
X   is our 'Xcellent audience here ;
Y   is for Year—come again please, next year.
Z   is the Zeal, which is shown by each helper
At the E. & W. Molesey Infant Welfare Centre.

Wellcome Images

Figure 1.1 East and West Molesey Infant Welfare Centre (Surrey) leaflet, 'Infant Welfare Centre ABC', circa 1930. Reproduced by permission of Wellcome Library, London.

Source: Wellcome Library, London

Feedback

1 The leaflet was targeted at the mothers of small children. We can tell this because of its focus on issues that relate to infants, but note also how it is addressed to mothers (under 'M') alone, and not mothers and fathers, a view of parenthood typical of the period. The focus on mothers reflected the idea that the health of the population could be bettered by improving the way in which children were raised. You may also

have noticed that other messages – not strictly related to the health of children – are communicated, such as 'E' for economy, 'F' for the future, and the rather stern sounding 'R' for rules. The leaflet is perhaps intended to inculcate other kinds of 'good' behaviours in the attending mothers, and is likely to be indicative of the middle-class values of those running the health centre.

2 It is, of course, difficult to know exactly what kind of an effect such a leaflet may have had on its audience. Some of the mothers may have welcomed the leaflet as an informative list of the kinds of facilities and advice they were likely to find at the centre. Others may have found the leaflet patronizing or condescending, especially if they did not share the values of those running the centre. Some mothers may have ignored the leaflet, and been more focused on the services that the centre offered at a time before free, comprehensive health care was widely available in Britain. Even today, as we will discuss below, efforts to promote good health do not always have the intended effect on their audience.

The development of health services

By the middle of the twentieth century, there were signs in many Western countries that preventing disease and promoting good health might have more of a role to play in health services. The Second World War helped to drive forward the development of centralized health systems in many European nations. In Britain, for example, early plans for the establishment of the National Health Service (NHS) appeared to emphasize disease prevention and health education. In 1944, a White Paper (draft legislation) on the NHS stated that the service aimed to: 'divorce the case of health from questions of personal means and other factors irrelevant to it: to provide the service free of charge ... and to encourage a new attitude to health – the easier obtaining of advice early, the promotion of good health rather than only the treatment of bad' (Ministry of Health, 1944).

The attention being directed to promoting good health, however, did seem to disappear once the NHS was established in 1948. Much greater emphasis was placed on treating sickness rather than promoting health. By the 1950s and 1960s, faith in high-tech medicine, and particularly so-called 'magic bullets' – specific drugs that could cure particular diseases – was at its height. There were some justified successes: due partly to drugs like antibiotics and also to vaccination programmes, epidemics of infectious diseases seemed to be a thing of the past, at least in the West. Ironically, this was a difficult period for public health medicine, as its old foes appeared to have been vanquished. Public health needed to find a new role.

Social medicine

One of the ways in which public health was able to revitalize itself was around the notion of social medicine. Social medicine developed in Britain during the 1930s and 1940s, and was concerned with what John Ryle (who was the first Professor of Social Medicine at Oxford University) described as the: 'whole economic, nutritional, occupational, educational and psychological opportunity or experience of the individual or community' (Ryle, 1948: 11–12). What Ryle and other proponents of social medicine were proposing was a much wider notion of health as a positive condition and not just the absence of disease. To this end, health professionals inspired by social medicine began to work with local communities to improve health.

Social medicine helped to change the focus of public health in other ways too, particularly by bringing the social sciences into health studies, and especially epidemiology. Research conducted during the 1940s and 1950s using epidemiological techniques identified specific behaviours, such as tobacco smoking and diet, as risk factors for developing diseases like lung cancer and coronary heart disease (Rothstein, 2003). In this way, social medicine was an important antecedent of many of the key aspects of what became known as the new public health.

Phase 3: 1970 to the present

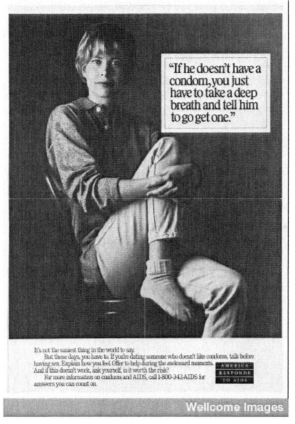

Figure 1.2 US Department of Health and Human Services poster from the 1990s. Reproduced by permission of Wellcome Library, London.

Source: Wellcome Library, London

Activity 1.4

Examine Figure 1.2, which is an AIDS prevention poster produced by the US Department of Health and Human Services in the 1990s, and then answer the following questions:

1 Who was this poster being targeted at?
2 What effect do you think this poster was designed to have on its audience?

Feedback

1 The poster was being targeted at heterosexual women. It is representative of a shift in ideas about who was likely to contract HIV from 'high-risk groups' – like gay men, intravenous drug users, and haemophiliacs – to the wider population of non-drug-using heterosexuals. The poster also tells us something about changing gender rela-tions, or at least the possibility that women may insist that a male sexual partner use a condom.
2 Clues to the intended effect of the poster appear in the text. 'Risk' is mentioned, and the campaign seems to be intended to influence individual behaviour in order to prevent the transmission of HIV and the development of AIDS. Risk, prevention, and a focus on individual behaviour were all crucial aspects of the new public health and the development of health promotion, as you will see in the next section. Again, as with the previous activity, it is difficult to know what affect such campaigns actually had on their intended audience. The lower than initially feared incidences of HIV/AIDS could be seen as evidence of the 'success' of such campaigns, but in many Western countries HIV/AIDS prevalence is now higher than it was in the late 1980s/early 1990s. Some critics have viewed such campaigns as potentially stigmatizing for people living with HIV/AIDS, an argument discussed in greater detail later in this chapter.

The new public health

Notions of risk, safety, prevention, and individual behaviour – as both a cause of disease and a way to combat it – were central to what was called the new public health. In part, this grew out of the challenge to conventional medicine. During the 1970s, biomedicine came under attack from two sides. First, the rising costs of health care, together with a weak global economy, made high-tech medicine increasingly expensive. At the same time, the shortcomings of health services in both high- and low-income countries were exposed, often through high-profile scandals about poor care. Second, theorists and researchers began to criticize the supposed victories of high-tech medicine. Particularly important here was the work of Thomas McKeown, Professor of Social Medicine at the University of Birmingham. McKeown argued that declining mortality rates at the end of the nineteenth century were the result not so much of medical advances, but of improved living standards and nutrition (McKeown, 1979). The McKeown thesis had an international impact. The influence of his work can be observed in a report produced by the Canadian Minister of Health, Marc LaLonde in 1974. The report, *A New Perspective on the Health of Canadians* (the LaLonde Report), acknowledged that improving living standards and public health measures were at least as important, if not more so, than biomedicine for the health of Canadians.

Health promotion and primary health care

Following the LaLonde Report, health promotion began to emerge as a specifically identifiable strand within public health (MacDougall, 2007). Health promotion differed from the more medicalized new public health by emphasizing the wider social influences upon collective and individual health. This can be seen in a number of developments globally. There were a series of initiatives introduced by the World Health Organization (WHO) in the late 1970s and 1980s that stressed the importance of promoting good health as well as combating disease. The 1978 Declaration of Alma Ata, for example, advocated a multidimensional approach to health and socio-economic development, and urged active community participation in health care and health education at every level, with a particular focus on primary health care (Cueto, 2004). In 1986, the Ottawa Charter for Health Promotion was introduced. This document shifted the focus of public health from disease prevention to 'capacity building for health'. This was tied through the work of the Pan American Health Organization (PAHO) and the European office of WHO (WHO Euro) to an approach that moved beyond health care to a commitment to social reform and equity (Kickbusch, 2003). To achieve this, specific targets were introduced, such as those developed by WHO Euro under the slogan 'Health for All by the Year 2000', which emphasized the importance of understanding health behaviours within their social context.

As part of this wider view of the determinants of health, by the late 1980s there were signs that the environment was returning to play a role in public health and health promotion. However, this took a slightly different form to the fixation with water and sanitation so much in evidence during the nineteenth century, at least in the higher-income countries. At the global and national levels, concern was expressed about resource depletion, pollution, and the creation of unhealthy environments and living conditions, especially in towns. There were moves to place the environment at the heart of attempts to secure good health for all. This can be seen in the Ottawa Charter for Health Promotion, which stated that: 'The fundamental conditions and resources for health are peace, shelter, education, food, income, a stable eco-system, sustainable resources, social justice and equity. Improvement in health requires a secure foundation in these basic prerequisites' (WHO, 1986).

The Ottawa Charter was also part of an attempt to encourage governments to take responsibility for creating environments that would make it possible for their populations to be healthy. But it was not only governments that took the lead here: there was some inter-sectoral cooperation, with the public and the community working together with government to make healthy environments possible. An example of this is the Healthy Cities Initiative. Launched in 1987, this project aimed to bypass national health ministries and localize health promotion, building a strong lobby at the local level (Petersen and Lupton, 1996).

The international health promotion movement initially retained a Canadian and European focus. In some countries such as the US, health education with its much longer history as a strategy was never replaced by health promotion. In other countries such as India, health promoting strategies had been used for longer but were not termed as such. Separate from health promotion, but with similarities, was another international movement that had its main influence in low-income countries. This was primary health care, driven forward after the Declaration of Alma Ata in 1978 (Berridge, 2010). The primary health care movement was concerned to find different ways of organizing basic health services in resource-poor countries. Early initiatives such as barefoot doctors in China and village health workers in Tanzania in the 1960s were important precursors. In Venezuela and Guatemala, ordinary people were trained to provide basic health care and Cuba also introduced a different model of health services. Later, through the influence of WHO and UNICEF, such approaches – in particular the use of community health workers – spread widely in what were then called 'developing countries'. There were heated debates about whether programmes should be 'horizontal' or 'vertical' (i.e. whether they should encompass wide service provision or simply focus on a few conditions and problems). The latter approach was more attractive to external donors (Walt, 2001). Only in the twenty-first century did concerns about chronic disease begin to surface in these countries.

Prevention and risk

Indeed, the development of health promotion at the global level had an impact on national and local public health policies too. A strong emphasis on disease prevention can be identified in national public health policy documents from this period, such as the UK's *Prevention and Health: Everybody's Business*, which we looked at in the opening exercise of this chapter (Department of Health, 1976). Such an emphasis on disease prevention was underpinned by epidemiology and the notion of risk. The case of smoking and lung cancer illustrates this well. The work of Doll and Hill (1954, 1956) identified smoking as a risk factor for developing lung cancer. Here was a behaviour – not an environmental factor – that was causing disease with the potential to affect the health of the population as a whole. As a result, a new public health agenda began to develop that stressed the need for behavioural change and for individuals to take responsibility for their own health. Advertising and the mass media were both used to promote good health and also encourage behavioural change. As you saw with the poster in Activity 1.4, emphasis was placed on preventing individuals from becoming sick.

In more recent years, it seems that the notion of risk has been broadened to include the risks that individuals or groups of individuals pose to the rest of the community, not just to their own health. Passive smoking is one example of this, with the relatively small risk posed by smokers to the health of others used to justify policies such as banning smoking in public places (Berridge, 2007). We can identify a subtle shift here: instead of focusing on individual behaviour and the risk that this poses to the health of the individual engaging in that behaviour, there is also an emphasis on the impact that behaviour has on the wider community. Is the idea of the risky individual giving way to that of protecting the safety of community?

Evidence for such a view can be found, for instance, in the recent reformulation of the UK's strategy on illegal drugs, which focuses more on reducing the crime associated with drug use than on providing treatment for individuals. Some critics fear that this could lead to a more punitive turn within the drugs field and in public health more broadly, as emphasis is placed on protecting the community from the risks posed by others. Such an approach adds weight to the arguments made by people who are critical of health promotion. By way of conclusion, we will examine some of these critiques and consider what these also say about the way health promotion has developed over the last 100 years or so.

Critiques of health promotion

In this section, we analyse three categories of attack made against health promotion: practical, structural, and surveillance. But first, complete Activity 1.5, which highlights some of these themes.

Activity 1.5

For some critics, health promotion still means health education only. In this activity, you will consider critiques of health education. Read the extracts below, which are taken from an article about health education by the British general practitioner and author James Le Fanu. Health education is a specific strand of health promotion that emphasizes learning to improve health. Once you have read the extracts, answer the questions that follow.

'Health education is an unexciting subject of marginal intellectual content. In essence, and this is certainly the overriding public impression, it takes the form of advertising slogans – or rather admonitions – which, were they complied with, are presumed to improve the health of the nation: don't drink and drive; wear a condom; smoking kills; eat healthily etc.' (p. 89)

'scientific attempts to evaluate health education promotions almost all show that it is actually very difficult to get people to change their behaviour by cajoling them to do so'. (p. 90)

'health education like any other branch of medicine is not without its "side effects" which would be – as with the case of drugs – acceptable if it worked, but unacceptable if it does not. These side effects would include frightening the public with misleading concepts about the risk of everyday life, the linking of pleasurable activities like eating and sex with disability and death. Do fish and chips clog up the arteries? Is unprotected casual heterosexual intercourse very risky? For those unfortunate enough to suffer from coronary heart disease or stroke, the health education message might have the "side effect" of blaming the victim where the sufferers believe that their misfortune is in large measure their own fault.' (p. 91)

'Over the last decade the Conservative government has enormously increased its direct involvement in the private lives of the nation through its resourcing of health education programmes. There are two sound reasons for regretting this development: it reinforces the ethos of the nanny state in which the notion that individuals are responsible for their own lives is marginalised; further, and this particularly applies to the AIDS campaign, it has been argued by, for example, the Chief Rabbi, the campaigns appear to endorse a moral message which sanctions casual sexual intercourse as long as it is performed "safely". To this extent health education can be said to have influenced the moral tone of the nation.' (pp. 91–2)

(Extracts from James Le Fanu (1994) Does health education work?, in J. Le Fanu (ed.) Preventionitis: The Exaggerated Claims of Health Promotion. London: Social Affairs Unit.)

1 Itemize the different concerns Le Fanu raises about health education.
2 How convincing are his arguments against health education?

Feedback

1 The concerns Le Fanu raises are: (a) Health education lacks an intellectual foundation and is instead based on telling people what to do. (b) There is little evidence to

show that health education works. (c) Health education has side-effects, including blaming the victim for his or her condition. (d) Health education undermines individual responsibility for health. (e) Health education may encourage 'immoral' behaviour, such as having casual sex.

2 Some of you will not have been convinced by Le Fanu's arguments. You may have noticed, for example, that in the extracts presented he does not cite any evidence for his contention that health education does not work. Le Fanu does draw on evidence to support his argument in the full article, such as studies of health education campaigns that have shown that behaviour is rarely changed by exposure to such material. But how do we know what causes an individual to change their behaviour? How long does it take for the effects of health promotion campaigns to be felt? You may also have picked up on the rather controversial tone of Le Fanu's writing. This may have made you feel less confident about his arguments. Yet, some of you could have found Le Fanu's statements more convincing. He does raise genuine concerns about whether or not health promotion works and its unintended effects. Regardless of whether or not you agree with Le Fanu, he does make some important points that health promoters need to take into account, issues that are discussed in more detail in the remainder of this chapter.

Practical

One of the key critiques directed at health promotion is that it simply does not work: it does not achieve the level of improvements in health it aims to. Critics like Le Fanu argue that the resources used on health promotion would be better spent on treating the sick rather than on preventing people getting ill. In practice, many national health systems are designed primarily to deal with the ill and tend to place less emphasis on disease prevention. Moreover, it could be argued, it makes sense when we only have finite resources to spend on health that these are best directed at those who are already ill. At the same time, from a political perspective, even if health promotion measures have an effect, it is likely that these can only be felt over a long period and are often difficult to measure.

Structural

A different kind of attack (often made by those on the left) is that health promotion fails to address the structural issues that underpin health. Insufficient attention, critics argue, is paid to the conditions that produce bad health such as poverty, poor housing, dangerous environments, and so on. Inequalities and health have made a re-appearance in health promotion in recent years, but many would suggest the insufficient attention is paid to this issue still (Marmot, 2004).

Another structural problem with health promotion is that by targeting individual behaviour and placing responsibility for health on individuals, it can have the effect of appearing to blame victims of disease for their condition (Crawford, 1977). In contrast, governments have been slow to target key actors such as the tobacco industry that produce the products that make people sick in the first place. Focusing on preventing sickness can also have the effect of increasing the stigma associated with being ill. As we saw with the HIV/AIDS prevention poster, such efforts state very clearly that being ill is an undesirable state, which increases the stigma attached to those who are unwell.

Surveillance

Finally, some see health promotion as a project that places large sections of the population under surveillance (Armstrong, 2008). Monitoring the health of the population can become a form of discipline. Exhorting people to behave in a proscribed way undermines individual agency and autonomy. Health promotion can thus become a tool of social control.

Conclusion

Now, whether or not you agree with these critiques, it is interesting that they echo many of the themes we have touched on in the long history of public health and health promotion. Surveillance, social control, stigmatization, whether to emphasize disease treatment or prevention are all themes that we have come across before. We have seen how the social determinants of health have often been ignored. In the nineteenth century, for example, poor living conditions were often to blame for sickness, but instead the working classes were pathologized and regarded as a source of disease. There has also long been a tendency to blame the victims of public health problems – we can see this in the late twentieth century and the emphasis on individual responsibility for health. It is also the case that public health and health promotion measures can be a form of social control. Intervention into people's lives, such as the introduction of health visitors in the early twentieth century, can have a disciplinary effect. Such issues, present in the past, are manifestly still with us in more recent attempts to safeguard public health and promote good health.

Summary

The history of health promotion illustrates some of the complexities and issues that health promotion continues to face today. Key points include:

- Health promotion as a specific discipline emerged in the 1970s.
- Health promotion was rooted in much earlier shifts within public health that stretch back to the nineteenth century and beyond.
- There is both continuity and change over time within public health and health promotion.
- Some issues appear, disappear, and re-appear, such as the environment.

References

Apple, R. (1987) Mothers and Medicine: A Social History of Infant Feeding, 1890–1950. Madison, WI: University of Wisconsin Press.

Armstrong, D. (2008) The rise of surveillance medicine, Sociology of Health and Illness, 17(3): 393–404.

Bashford, A. and Levine, P. (eds.) (2010) The Oxford Handbook of the History of Eugenics. Oxford: Oxford University Press.

Berridge, V. (2007) Marketing Health: Smoking and the Discourse of Public Health in Britain, 1945–2000. Oxford: Oxford University Press.

Berridge, V. (2010) Historical and policy approaches, in Y. Coombes and M. Thorogood (eds.) *Evaluating Health Promotion: Practice and Methods* (3rd edn.). Oxford: Oxford University Press.

Chadwick, E. (1843) *Report on the Sanitary Condition of the Labouring Population of Great Britain: A Supplementary Report on the Results of a Special Inquiry into the Practice of Interment in Towns.* London: W. Clownes.

Crawford, R. (1977) You are dangerous to your health: the ideology and politics of victim blaming, *International Journal of Health Services*, 7(4): 663–80.

Cueto, M. (2004) The origins of primary health care and selective primary health care, *American Journal of Public Health*, 94(11): 1864–74.

Davies, C. (1988) The health visitor as mother's friend: a woman's place in public health, 1900–14, *Social History of Medicine*, 1(1): 39–59.

de Vries, J. (1984) *European Urbanization 1500–1800.* London: Methuen.

Department of Health (1976) *Prevention and Health: Everybody's Business.* London: HMSO.

Doll, R. and Hill, A.B. (1954) The mortality of doctors in relation to their smoking habits, *British Medical Journal*, ii: 1451–5. (Reprinted 2004 in *British Medical Journal*, 328(7455: 1529–33.)

Doll, R. and Hill, A.B. (1956) Lung cancer and other causes of death in relation to smoking: a second report on the mortality of British doctors, *British Medical Journal*, 2(5001): 1071–81.

Donajgrodzki, A.P. (ed.) (1977) *Social Control in Nineteenth Century Britain.* London: Croom Helm.

Durbach, N. (2005) *Bodily Matters: The Anti-Vaccination Movement in England, 1853–1907.* Durham, NC: Duke University Press.

Dyhouse, C. (1978) Working-class mothers and infant mortality in England, 1895–1914, *Journal of Social History*, 12(2): 248–67.

Hamlin, C. (1998) *Public Health and Social Justice in the Age of Chadwick, Britain 1800–1854.* Cambridge: Cambridge University Press.

Hennock, E.P. (1998) Vaccination policy against smallpox, 1835–1914: a comparison of England with Prussia and Imperial Germany, *Social History of Medicine*, 11(1): 49–71.

Jones, G. (1986) *Social Hygiene in Twentieth Century Britain.* Beckenham: Croom Helm.

Kickbusch, I. (2003) The contribution of the World Health Organization to a new public health and health promotion, *American Journal of Public Health*, 93(3): 383–8.

LaLonde, M. (1974) *A New Perspective on the Health of Canadians* (the LaLonde Report). Ottawa, Ontario: Minister of Supply and Services.

Le Fanu, J. (1994) Does health education work?, in J. Le Fanu (ed.) *Preventionitis: The Exaggerated Claims of Health Promotion:* London: Social Affairs Unit.

MacDougall, H. (2007) Reinventing public health: a new perspective on the health of Canadians and its international impact, *Journal of Epidemiology and Community Health*, 61: 955–9.

Marmot, M. (2004) *Status Syndrome: How Your Social Standing Directly Affects Your Health.* London: Bloomsbury.

McKeown, T. (1979) *The Role of Medicine.* Oxford: Blackwell.

Melosi, M. (2000) *The Sanitary City: Urban Infrastructure in America from Colonial Times to the Present.* Baltimore, MD: Johns Hopkins University Press.

Ministry of Health (1944) *A National Health Service.* Cmnd. 6502. London: HMSO.

Petersen, A. and Lupton, D. (1996) *The New Public Health: Health and Self in an Age of Risk.* London: Sage.

Porter, D. (1999) *Health, Civilisation and the State: A History of Public Health from Ancient to Modern Times.* Abingdon: Routledge.

Rothstein, W. (2003) *Public Health and the Risk Factor: A History of an Uneven Medical Revolution.* Rochester, NY: University of Rochester Press.

Ryle, J.A. (1943) Social medicine, its meaning and scope, *British Medical Journal*, ii: 633–6.

Ryle, J.A. (1948) *Changing Disciplines.* London: Oxford University Press.

Snow, S. (2002) Commentary: Sutherland, Snow and water: the transmission of cholera in the nineteenth century, *International Journal of Epidemiology*, 31(5): 908–11.

Walt, G. (2001) Health care in the developing world, 1974–2001, in C. Webster (ed.) *Caring for Health: History and Diversity.* Buckingham: Open University Press.

Wohl, A. (1983) *Endangered Lives: Public Health in Victorian Britain*. London: Methuen.

Worboys, M. (2000) *Spreading Germs: Disease Theories and Medical Practice in Britain, 1865–1900*. Cambridge: Cambridge University Press.

World Health Organization (WHO) (1978) *Declaration of Alma-Ata*. Available at: http://www.who.int/publications/almaata_declaration_en.pdf.

World Health Organization (WHO) (1986) *The Ottawa Charter for Health Promotion*. Available at: http://www.who.int/healthpromotion/conferences/previous/ottawa/en/ [accessed 18 October 2012].

2 Social construction of health and health promotion

Sara Cooper and Nicki Thorogood

Overview

The aim of this chapter is to introduce you to social constructionism as a particular conceptual framework and how it might be applied to the concepts of health and health promotion. First, we provide a brief introduction to social constructionism and how such a conceptual framework shapes our understanding and thinking about the social world. Second, we examine how a social constructionist conceptual framework might be applied to health. Here we introduce two different intellectual strands of a social constructionist stance towards health and illness, exploring how, in slightly different ways, they have both made a major contribution to our understanding of the context-dependent dimensions of illness and disease entities. Third, we explore what implications a social constructionist conceptual framework has for health promotion. We demonstrate how it might help us to think critically about the concepts, categories, and definitions used within health promotion programmes, which could enable the practice of health promotion to be more self-aware, self-critical, and accountable. Applying a social constructionist conceptual framework to health promotion, however, takes us further than this. It also forces us to look critically at the whole health promotion endeavour itself; to consider what role it plays and what consequences it might have in society more generally. An analysis at this level encourages us to think about health promotion's potential to act as a form of social regulation and whether it can be uncritically regarded as 'good'.

Learning objectives

After reading this chapter, you will be able to:

- understand social constructionism as a particular conceptual framework
- appreciate how a social constructionist conceptual framework might be applied to the concept of health and medical knowledge
- identify the implications social constructionism has for health promotion theory and practice

Key terms

Disciplinary power: A modern and more concealed form of power that works through systems of knowledge and practice, which, by creating standards of 'normality' and 'abnormality', induces people to constantly examine and adjust themselves and others according to such norms.

Discourse: Bodies of language, knowledge, and practice that constitute the very things they appear to describe.

Normative: Behaviours and practices that are viewed as 'normal' or 'correct' in a particular social context.

Phenomenology: A qualitative research paradigm, derived from the writings of philosophers such as Husserl and Buber, which focuses on the lived and subjective experience of phenomena. It seeks to describe and appreciate how people themselves understand and give meaning to their own experiences.

Semiotics: The study of signs and symbols which aims to deconstruct their coded meanings. It includes signs and symbols in any medium or sensory modality (e.g. words, images, sounds, gestures, and objects).

Social constructionism: A critical conceptual framework which understands things that are generally thought to be exclusively natural as being socially produced.

What is social constructionism?

Social constructionism is a conceptual framework that understands things – generally thought to be exclusively natural – as being socially produced. Its emphasis is on how meanings of phenomena are not inherent in the phenomena themselves, but are created through interaction and dialogue within a particular historically situated social context (Gergen, 1999). Such a perspective rejects the suggestion that there is an objective, single, and pre-existing 'truth' that is 'out there', waiting to be discovered. Rather, social constructionists argue that social reality, and knowledge about it, is multiple and always context-dependent, and is the product of social, historical, political, and cultural processes (Berger and Luckmann, 1966). Understandings of phenomena may therefore vary over time, and experiences may be assigned different meanings across different social groups and settings. To take a simple example, child labour was considered perfectly normal in Britain during the early nineteenth century whereas now it is subject to rigorous legislation.

As a particular approach to human enquiry, social constructionism invariably has a critical agenda (Burr, 2003), since it seeks to question taken-for-granted knowledge about the social world and how we categorize it, which proclaims itself (sometimes subtly and sometimes not so subtly) to be self-evident truth. Such a perspective attempts to deconstruct the terms we use routinely; interrogating their absolute and inevitable appearance. It seeks to unpack the assumptions, ideologies, and power relations that are embedded in, and reinforced by, the categories that are employed. It asks questions such as: What are the processes by which phenomena become classified in particular ways? Who has the power to produce legitimate classifications? And what are the consequences of such classifications?

Thus, for example, a social constructionist perspective contends that 'gender' is socially constructed and as such the roles, abilities, and temperaments that are assigned to a particular gender are shaped by commonly accepted norms about what a man or woman should be like or how they ought to behave rather than reflecting inherent truths found in nature. A social constructionist perspective might also emphasize how dominant constructions of femininity and masculinity have frequently served to naturalize and justify gender inequality. For example, it has been argued that the common construction of womanhood as quintessentially caring and nurturing has contributed to the concentration of women in part-time and lower paid employment, and reduced their opportunities for training and promotion (Charles, 1993).

Similarly, social constructionists argue that the category 'race' is more of a socially produced notion than the expression of any major biological essences. They claim that apparently 'natural' racial taxonomies act to reify 'race' as a predetermined reality and to essentialize racial differences that have in turn been used to exploit and oppress certain groups. For example, there is a long history of constructing black Africans as genetically distinct and primitive, which has been employed to support political projects such as slavery, imperialism, anti-immigration policy, and the eugenics movement (Williams et al., 1994; Bhopal, 1997; Krieger, 2000).

Activity 2.1

In this activity you will apply the framework of social constructionism to your own examples. Pause for a moment and try to think of any examples from your own knowledge and experience where accepted social categories have come into question.

Feedback

You might, for example, have recalled the way apparently 'real' racial classifications in South Africa changed after the end of the apartheid era. What does this say about the 'nature' of racial categories? Or you might have considered how the acceptance of women as being suitable for roles such as surgeons or for military duty has now changed (although it is still commonly held that women are not suitable for frontline fighting). What views of the 'nature' of women does this imply? Or you might have reflected on how it was once an uncontested truth that the earth was flat.

The social construction of health and illness

Over the last 50 years, the social construction of health has become a significant perspective within the sociology of health and illness, and has made a major contribution to our understanding of the context-dependent dimensions of illness (Bury, 1986; Lupton, 2000). Although there are various intellectual strands within a social constructionist approach to illness, two broad threads can be identified that have addressed this topic slightly differently.

The social construction of 'lay' understandings and experiences of health and illness

The first tradition, which draws heavily on interpretive sociological perspectives, particularly phenomenology, takes the subjective meaning and experience of health and illness seriously. Here, the focus is on what are termed 'lay' people (as opposed to 'experts' who have training in specific practices, skills, and academic disciplines) and their personal understandings and enactments of well-being. Researchers in this tradition have addressed questions such as: How do 'lay' people understand health and illness? How do they make sense of and manage the onset of disease? What meanings are given to health-related behaviours? And how is health maintained in the lay sphere?

Such research has demonstrated that conceptualizations of health are neither universal nor given. Rather, they are context-bound, influenced by prevailing ideologies and mediated by the wider milieu in which people live, such as their cultural context, structural and geographic location, social identity, and personal biography. Understandings of health are at once individual and social and infinitely varied. What is defined as unhealthy in one culture may be celebrated in another. For example, some cultural groups might regard women's menstruation as a sign of disease, connoting moral and spiritual uncleanliness. As a consequence, during menses various taboos might be observed in areas such as clothing, bathing, food, social interaction, and sexual relationship. Other groups, however, might see menstruation as a sign of health and fertility for women. Both sets of practices are perceived as 'natural' and 'right' within their own societies and there will be sanctions invoked for any breaches. From a social constructionist perspective, we can regard these 'truths' as socially produced knowledge.

Similarly, conceptualizations about health and illness are not stable over time, but shift and adapt as prevailing social and political ideologies change. For example, Crawford (1994, 2006) tracks the radical changes that have occurred in understandings of health in Western societies over the last 200 years. He highlights how, before the eighteenth century, health was more likely to be perceived as part of an inclusive 'good fortune' and the outcome of good living, ritual observance or divine grace. As Europe and America modernized and industrialized, health emerged as something that could be achieved and was seen as an essential foundation of character and good citizenship. Understandings of health thus increasingly began to reflect the values of capitalism and individualism, being imbued with notions of individual autonomy, self-control, self-discipline, and willpower.

Research within this tradition has also demonstrated how health-related behaviours and choices are embedded in socio-economic structures and cultural contexts. For example, research in Canada (Shoveller et al., 2004), the UK (Thorogood, 1995), and South Africa (Wood and Foster, 1995; Shefer and Foster, 2001) has revealed that sexual practices have significant social, personal, and cultural meanings which often have very little to do with health. Sexual behaviour and related decisions in the context of people's everyday lives are frequently influenced by discourses such as those pertaining to desire, intimacy, trust, morality, and danger. Similarly, research into the reproductive choices among HIV-positive women in many African countries also demonstrates how such decisions are frequently shaped by social and cultural norms and expectations, rather than health concerns. The strong social and cultural norms around fertility in many African societies, which can result in childless women being marginalized and even facing death, has been shown to be a major influence in many HIV-positive women's decisions to have children (Aka-Dago-Akribi et al., 1997; Dyer et al., 2002; Myer and Morroni, 2005). Research into women and smoking has similarly illustrated the socially and contextually entrenched nature of health-related behaviours. It has been found that for many working-class women, smoking promotes an emotional sense of well-being and may enhance social capital. As Graham (1987: 55) concludes from her study of women caring for pre-school children in low-income families in Britain, 'Smoking acts as both a luxury and a necessity when material and human resources are stretched ... In a lifestyle stripped of new clothes, make-up, hair-dressing, travel by bus and evenings out, smoking can become an important symbol of one's participation in an adult consumer culture.'

A final major line of research within this tradition has examined the personal and social meanings of illness at the experiential level, and explored how illness is managed within the social contexts that people inhabit. Such research has highlighted how the experience of illness is socially constructed, contingent on how the sufferer comes to make sense of, and live with, their illness, and reclaim a sense of self. People may assign different meanings to their distress and suffering, depending on, for example, their personal and social relationships, class, gender, religious and cultural beliefs. As such, the everyday enactment and experience of illness is endowed with subjective meaning and is infinitely varied. The ways in which people actively determine the boundaries of their illness, and their identity in relationship to those parameters, has been demonstrated in the case of various specific illnesses including depression (Karp, 1996), epilepsy (Schneider and Conrad, 1983), schizophrenia (Schulze and Angermeyer, 2003), rheumatoid arthritis (Fagerlind et al., 2010), diabetes (Peyrot et al., 1987), asthma (Adams et al., 1997), and HIV/AIDS (Davies, 1997; Ezzy, 2000; Klitzman and Beyer, 2003).

Activity 2.2

This activity encourages you to reflect on the impact of taking lay beliefs and experiences into account when designing health promotion interventions. Imagine, for example, that you have been asked to design a health promotion intervention to change eating habits in a population of adolescents. How might taking into account young people's 'lay' beliefs about, and experiences of, food, diet, and health affect your plans? Jot down a few ideas for a setting you are familiar with. Ask yourself, what assumptions are the 'health experts' making about this group? How might they differ from the views of others – for example, non-health professionals (youth workers, church leaders, educationalists, politicians, etc.) or young people? Can you think of examples of this from your own professional, or lay, experiences?

Feedback

Health professionals may feel that they know what a desirable outcome is in terms of young people's eating habits and that they have simply to enable these to be adopted. Thus, perhaps, the 'professional' intervention may be no more than a socially constructed norm about what is desirable, without taking into account other aspects of the social world that may be as, if not more, important for this target group as 'good health'. This might include, for example, ideas about what constitutes 'attractiveness' for young men and young women, or their expectations of physical health and well-being.

Note also that 'young people' do not form a homogeneous group and appropriate interventions may vary with the prevailing social norms such as those relating to socio-economic class, gender or ideas about autonomy. Professionals may also wrongly assume that all of these social variables are pertinent to all young people at all times.

The social construction of medical knowledge and disease entities

A second intellectual strand within the constructionist approach to illness that draws heavily on the writings of Michel Foucault (1977) has contributed to our understanding of the socially constructed nature of health, albeit in a slightly different vein. What we might call the Foucauldian tradition looks critically at medical knowledge and disease entities, interrogating how and why particular signs and symptoms get labelled as medically legitimate illnesses (Jordanova, 1995; Turner, 1995; Bunton and Petersen, 1997; Lupton, 1997).

According to Foucault (1977), expert knowledge about 'health' and 'disease' is not an objective 'discovery' of a 'given' biological reality that simply exists in nature. Rather, accepted illness categories or disease entities are products of medical discourse that is shaped by social, cultural, and political reasoning and practices. Certain behaviours and experiences are conferred the status of medical conditions or illnesses within a particular time and place, and for Foucault, such constructions are a principal form of power in modern societies. For example, when a group of symptoms is categorized within medical discourse as 'tuberculosis', it does not mean that this entity exists independently 'out there', but rather it has been defined or labelled as such within a particular social, historical, and political context.

The socially constructed nature of disease entities is clearly illustrated by the fact that disease vocabularies and categories are not stable; boundaries and meanings of illness are perpetually contested, negotiated, and redefined over time. Throughout history there are examples of diagnoses and disease categories that have disappeared from clinical textbooks, and new 'diseases' are frequently being 'discovered' and named. The constant revision of the International Statistical Classification of Diseases and Related Health Problems (ICD) and Diagnostic and Statistical Manual of Mental Disorders (DSM) is testament to this.

Scholars within this Foucauldian tradition have demonstrated that these shifts in the classifications of disease entities are less the outcome of medico-scientific evidence and diagnostic procedures becoming more advanced or accurate, and more the product of changing social practices and political ideas. It is also stressed that decisions concerning what constitutes a disease are not value-neutral, but are mediated by political and moral values and ideologies that prevail within society. Illness categories therefore have a strong evaluative agenda, often supporting the interests of those groups in power, and reinforcing existing social structures.

For example, until the mid-1980s, homosexuality was defined and categorized in the International Classification of Diseases (widely used within the USA and Western Europe) as a medical condition requiring treatment. It is not difficult to see how this official medical diagnosis occurred within the context of powerful socio-political forces that were against variations from the traditional heterosexual dyad that prevailed for much of the twentieth century (Hare-Mustin and Marecek, 1997; Smith et al., 2004). Similarly, a number of scholars have demonstrated how the development of a host of diseases associated with sexuality and reproduction during the nineteenth century were intimately shaped by patriarchal structures and contemporary social mores about women's 'proper' place in society (Jacobus et al., 1990; Ussher, 1991,

1996). Nineteenth-century illnesses such as neurasthenia and hysteria were attributed to supposed aberrations of the reproductive system, and women were therefore encouraged to concentrate on dulling the mind, intellectually and emotionally, to enable the functions of their body to ensue unhindered by mental obstruction.

To summarize this section on the social construction of health, unlike a medical model of illness which assumes that diseases are universal and stable across time and place, a social constructionist approach emphasizes how all meanings, experiences, and definitions are produced by social interactions, shared cultural traditions, shifting frameworks of knowledge, and relations of power. All of this is not to deny the realities of pain and suffering, or to say that people do not experience bodily or mental distress. A social constructionist perspective emphasizes, however, that these experiences, and how we label them, are not just a result of medico-scientific procedures, but also the product of historical, social, and political processes.

Implications for health promotion

What are the implications of a social constructionist perspective, both generally and more specifically in relation to health, for health promotion? An appreciation that lay meanings of health and health-related behaviours are inextricably context-bound and socially shaped is crucial for making health education and promotion campaigns relevant and responsive to the target groups' lived experiences and subjective understandings. This is essential both for bringing the person's needs back into health promotion as an end in itself and for the potential effectiveness of health promotion programmes. Encouraging people to modify their lifestyles and adopt healthier ways of living in isolation from the social context in which these arise and develop meaning is somewhat artificial and may prove to be ineffective. For example, health promotion messages that simply advise people to stop smoking or practise safer sex will remain ineffective if the decisions surrounding these behaviours carry social, cultural, and symbolic meanings other than those which pertain to health, which they invariably do. The work of Holland et al. (1990a, 1990b), Wilton and Aggleton (1990), Campbell (2003), and Bernays and Rhodes (2009) has clearly demonstrated this in the case of HIV/AIDS. Campaigns and interventions that conceptualize health behaviour denuded of social meaning are likely to increase victim blaming and stigma, and have limited success.

Furthermore, a social constructionist perspective within a more Foucauldian tradition is vital for sensitizing health promoters to the importance of thinking critically about the concepts and categories that are employed. Such a perspective reminds us how all definitions and classifications are produced by people, in a particular time and place, and are thus always imbued with particular norms, assumptions, and social forces. It encourages us to think about how the problem is defined or framed in the first place, how it was developed, and what the consequences might be of adopting such a paradigm. This is essential if the practice of health promotion is to be self-aware, self-critical, and accountable. Indeed, social constructionist critiques have been instrumental in articulating the frequently hidden ideologies embedded in many health promotion campaigns.

For example, attacks have been levied on the uncritical use of racial categories within many HIV/AIDS health education and promotion programmes in Africa, and how this has produced devastatingly racist stereotypes of African people and their sexualities (Sabatier, 1988; Crewe and Aggleton, 2003; Stillwaggon, 2003; Campbell, 2004). Similarly, social constructionists have demonstrated how the norms and values attributed to target groups within many HIV/AIDS health education and promotion strategies in the

UK have supported gender stereotypes (Holland et al., 1990c; Wilton, 1997) and reinforced homophobia and discriminary practices (Treichler, 1989; Watney, 1989). Another example, this time from the USA, is the US Government's health information campaigns as part of the on-going so-called 'war on obesity', which has promoted the message that weight loss is simply a matter of self-control. In a context in which weight and health have been connected to patriotism and morality in the USA, such campaigns have been shown to have significantly increased the stigma associated with being overweight and obese (Garcia, 2007). A final example is from the UK, where during the 1980s health education campaigns directed at 'ethnic minorities', such as those concerned with rickets, surma, and antenatal care, were seen to have contributed to the construction of racist stereotypes and the augmentation of institutional racism (Sheiham and Quick, 1982; Pearson, 1986).

Semiotics

As demonstrated above, a social constructionist perspective helps us to think critically about the meanings embedded within health promotion activities. Meaning, however, is not only embedded within written or spoken language, but is also inserted within other mediums such as images, sounds, gestures, and objects. Here a strand of social constructionism, known as semiotics, can be very useful, as many health promotion initiatives use images as a key form of communication. Semiotics is the study of signs and symbols, especially systems of communication, in an attempt to deconstruct their coded meanings (Chandler, 2008). It includes signs and symbols in any medium or sensory modality (e.g. words, images, sounds, gestures, and objects). Semiotics is based on the assumption that signs do not just 'convey' meanings, but also constitute a medium in which meanings are *constructed*. The objective is therefore to reveal how certain values, attitudes, and beliefs are supported or silenced within particular signs and symbols. Meaning might be divided into two levels within semiotics: denotation and connotation. 'Denotation' refers to the more definitional, 'literal' or 'obvious' meaning of a sign, whereas 'connotation' refers to the deeper socio-cultural, political, economic, and 'personal' associations (ideological, socio-political, emotional, etc.) of the sign.

Activity 2.3

In this activity you will analyse a health promotion intervention using a social constructionist and semiotic perspective. Consider the poster shown as Figure 2.1. Who do you think it is aimed at (and what makes you think that)? What does its location in an urban town in a Sub-Saharan African country suggest to you (and why)? What wider message might it be hoping to convey (how does it make you 'know' this)? Now you have briefly deconstructed this poster using discourse analysis and semiotics ask yourself: In whose interests is this poster being displayed? What is absent from it? What assumptions are implicit in it? Does it tell you anything about wider social norms?

Feedback

The method of discourse analysis and semiotics takes text and image and 'deconstructs' their explicit and implicit meanings. Where words and image act together, as in

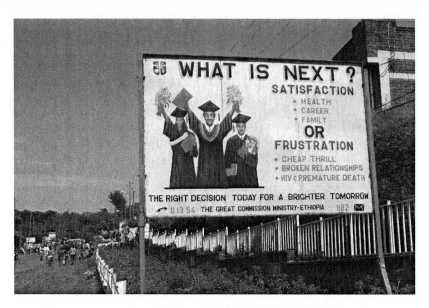

Figure 2.1 A government HIV awareness poster on the roadside in Jimma Town, Ethiopia (photograph taken in 2006). Reproduced by permission of Sasha Andrews, Wellcome Images.

Source: Sasha Andrews, Wellcome Images (image no. N0032219: http://wellcomeimages.org/)

the poster, both the image and the text constitute the object of the analysis. A semiotic approach asks us to consider two levels of meaning in an image, its denotation, or its literal meaning. In this case it is one woman and two men, each holding onto a bunch of flowers and a book, and wearing formal academic dress.

A second level is its connotation; that is all the other attributes that are implied and which depend on the system of values and meanings we bring to it. For example, in this case, we might 'know' that these three individuals are graduating students because of the academic gowns and caps worn. We might also infer a sense of hope and optimism through the images of flowers and arms raised in the air.

Without the text we may not be able to 'know' what wider message this image seeks to convey. However both the literal meaning of the text and the way it is presented give us 'clues'. We might 'read into it' that these three students are confronted with deciding what their future will hold, a decision that is seen to consist of only two options: 'satisfaction' or 'frustration'. The 'right decision' to make for a 'brighter tomorrow' is represented in no uncertain terms as one which embraces health, career and family.

You might have wondered why this campaign is focused on students, rather than other age-groups. You might have speculated on the apparent markers of 'satisfaction' and 'frustration', and why certain notions are provided and contrasted, and not others. You might also have questioned whether one's future is something that can be 'decided-upon' and 'chosen'.

This might suggest wider social norms about what it means to be happy and successful in the world, intimately related to notions of personal health, occupational achievements and familial obligations, and embroiled with ideals of individual agency. Or, conversely, a more benign reading might see it as depicting young people as able to make independent and responsible decisions about their futures. The text plus images might also lead you to 'know', without the inclusion of the country name, that the poster is situated in Africa, as all the people depicted are black and the language 'style' of the text and the reference to HIV might reasonably suggest this. There are also no white people shown, and this, situated in many other settings might be deemed inappropriate, exclusive or even racist.

Another 'layer' of analysis might have you wondering whether there are any common factors between those people that 'read' it one way and those that 'read' it another, and, if so, how these differences might have come about.

Health promotion as a form of disciplinary power

These multi-level layers of analysis show how a social constructionist perspective for health promotion can take us further than only thinking critically about the accepted concepts, categories, and definitions used, and their embedded assumptions within health promotion programmes. It also urges us to look critically at the whole health promotion endeavour itself, and what role it plays – and what consequences it might have – in society more generally. A social constructionist perspective of health promotion seeks to ask questions about the broader goals and aims of health promotion, and whether it can be uncritically regarded as 'good'. Analyses at this level have drawn attention to health promotion's propensity to act as a form of social regulation (Armstrong, 1983; Thorogood, 1992; Nettleton and Bunton, 1995).

Here, we are brought back to the work of Foucault, and his ideas concerning modern forms of power. As touched on earlier, Foucault saw medical discourse as a principal form of power in modern societies. To understand this fully, and how health promotion might function as a type of social control, one needs to appreciate how a Foucauldian approach conceptualizes the operation of power in contemporary, liberal democracies. According to Foucault (1980, 1984), modern forms of power operate differently to traditional forms of power. In this view, traditional power is conceptualized as 'sovereign' and is seen as regressive and coercive, whereas modern configurations of power are exercised in much more diffuse and typically covert ways, functioning at the micro-level of individuals. Such modern forms of power, or what Foucault terms 'disciplinary power', function through social systems of knowledge and practice that create standards pertaining to 'normality' and 'abnormality', 'healthy' and 'unhealthy'. It operates through providing guidelines about how people should understand, conduct, regulate, and experience their bodies, minds, and subjectivities. The objective of such modern forms of power is thus to produce 'obedient' subjects or 'disciplined objects', which constantly examine and adjust themselves and others to fit the norms and ideals it prescribes.

From this perspective, through the establishment of norms regarding appropriate and healthy experiences and behaviour, the programmes and technologies of health promotion can be seen as a form of disciplinary power and social regulation. As Wilbraham (2004: 460) articulates:

> There are now pervasive networks of health authorities, techniques and practices that seek to shape the conduct of individuals and populations. For example, think of: medical insurance, self-help books, advice columns, hygiene instructions at schools, yoga, aerobics classes, safer sex techniques, examinations in a doctor's consulting room, diabetic diets and so on.

Through all of these programmes, health promotion discourse and practice results in an increasingly all-encompassing network of surveillance and observation. Such discourse has penetrated the minds of lay people, who more and more willingly draw upon prevailing health promotion vocabularies to interpret their own experiences, and reflect upon, monitor, and think about themselves. People ever more frequently make particular choices and adopt specific behaviours that are expected by health promotion discourses. Indeed, seemingly subjective choices and activities – food and eating, sleeping, leisure, aspects of bodily maintenance, sexual behaviour – are increasingly becoming amenable to personal monitoring and regulation. Ultimately, as people become progressively caught within the discourses of health promotion, they actively and readily seek to develop their lifestyles, bodies, minds, and subjectivities in accordance with the prevailing truth configurations of it. Indeed, this is a fundamental component of modern forms of power, which seek to:

> Establish voluntary practices by means of which individuals not only create for themselves the rules of conduct, but also endeavour to transform themselves, to modify their unique being … and [thus] come to think of his own being when he recognises himself as mad, when he regards himself as ill, when he thinks of himself as a living being, working and talking, when he judges and punishes himself as criminal.
>
> (Foucault, 2004: 709)

This all may seem to imply that health promotion is a coercive and repressive enterprise. On the contrary, Foucault's analysis of 'disciplinary power' emphasizes that such power is not necessarily negative or oppressive, or for the purpose of coercion and constraint (Lupton, 1997). Indeed, he argued that the very seductiveness of power in modern societies is that it is productive rather than confining:

> What makes power hold good, what makes it accepted, is simply the fact that it doesn't only weigh on us a force that says no, but that it traverses and produces things, it induces pleasure, forms of knowledge, produces discourse. It needs to be considered as a productive network which runs through the whole social body, much more than as a negative instance whose function is repression.
>
> (Foucault, 1984: 61)

As such, it is exactly because health promotion attempts to improve our lives and make us healthier beings that it is able to wield such immense power.

Activity 2.4

In this activity, you will explore your own personal health-related behaviour from a social constructionist perspective using a 'Diary of your day'. Make a list of the things you do on a typical day, listing all the activities in which you participate (voluntarily) that currently form part of the 'health promotion' project.

Feedback

Your diary might have included: cleaning your teeth, taking a vitamin tablet, limiting the amount of coffee you drink, feeling guilty (self-monitoring) because you have used the escalator rather than the stairs or driven rather than walked to your destination, reading the label on the sandwich you bought for lunch, deciding how to prepare your evening meal in a healthy way, and so on. Have a look through these and ask yourself how would this list have looked to someone 50 or 100 years ago? How might it look in the future (5, 10, 20 or 100 years from now)? In this way, we might be able to 'see' how knowledge about what is 'normal' and 'desirable', and the assumptions and behaviours that are predicated on it, can easily change over time. Pause for a moment, does this change the way you feel about your daily activities? Does it make you feel more, or perhaps less, inclined to 'discipline' yourself in this way?

Summary

This chapter has introduced you to social constructionism as a particular critical, theoretical orientation, which stresses the socially produced nature of reality and knowledge about it. We have outlined how such a conceptual framework might be applied to the notion of health in two slightly different ways. First, situated within a more interpretive sociological perspective, social constructionism emphasizes how conceptualizations and experiences of health and health-related behaviours are intrinsically context-bound, deeply influenced by prevailing ideologies and mediated by the wider milieu in which people live. From a slightly more critical, Foucauldian perspective, a social constructionist stance emphasizes how medical knowledge and disease entities do not simply reflect 'given' biological realities, but are produced by medical discourse. This discourse is shaped fundamentally by social, cultural, and political reasoning and practices.

We then looked at the implications of such a perspective for health promotion. We demonstrated how a social constructionist approach might assist with bringing the 'person' back into health promotion activities, which could in turn enhance the potential effectiveness of interventions. Such a perspective also helps us to think critically about the concepts, categories, and definitions used within health promotion programmes. This is important for minimizing the potential perpetuation and reinforcement of particular forms of social and structural inequality and oppression through health promotion discourse and practice. Finally, we attempted to introduce the idea that when viewed though a social constructionist lens, the wider goals and aims of health promotion are brought into question. In this light, one is urged to consider how health promotion discourse and practice may act as a form of social regulation, and whether it might necessarily be regarded as 'good'. Ultimately, however helpful and beneficial the discourses and practices of health promotion might be, we have hopefully demonstrated that it remains an immense form of power that transforms how we think, controls what we desire, and modifies how we behave. The question we need to consider is what other ways of being, and what alternative choices, are potentially being silenced by the normalizing tendencies of health promotion discourse and practice?

References

Adams, S., Pill, R. and Jones, A. (1997) Medication, chronic illness and identity: the perspective of people with asthma, *Social Science and Medicine*, 45: 189–201.

Aka-Dago-Akribi, H., Desgrees Du Lou, A., Msellati, P., Doussou, R. and Welffens-Ekra, C. (1997) Issues surrounding reproductive choice for women living with HIV in Abidjan, Cote d'Ivoire, *Reproductive Health Matters*, 7(13): 20–9.

Armstrong, D. (1983) *Political Anatomy of the Body: Medical Knowledge in Britain in the Twentieth Century*. Cambridge: Cambridge University Press.

Berger, P. and Luckmann, T. (1966) *The Social Construction of Reality*. New York: Doubleday.

Bernays, S. and Rhodes, T. (2009) Experiencing uncertain HIV treatment delivery in a transitional setting: qualitative study, *AIDS Care*, 21(3): 315–21.

Bhopal, R.S. (1997) Is research into ethnicity and health racist, unsound, or important science?, *British Medical Journal*, 314(7096): 1751–6.

Bunton, R. and Petersen, A. (eds.) (1997) *Foucault, Health and Medicine*. London: Routledge.

Burr, V. (2003) *Social Constructionism* (2nd edn.). London: Routledge.

Bury, M.R. (1986) Social constructionism and the development of medical sociology, *Sociology of Health and Illness*, 8: 137–69.

Campbell, C. (2003) *'Letting Them Die': Why HIV/AIDS Prevention Programmes Fail*. Oxford: James Currey.

Campbell, C. (2004) The role of collective action in the prevention of HIV/AIDS in South Africa, in D. Hook (ed.) *Critical Psychology*. Cape Town: UCT Press.

Chandler, D. (2008) *Semiotics for Beginners*. Available at: http://www.aber.ac.uk/media/Documents/S4B/sem06.html [accessed 18 October 2012].

Charles, N. (1993) *Gender Divisions and Social Change*. Brighton: Harvester.

Crawford, R. (1994) The boundaries of the self and the unhealthy other: reflections on health, culture and AIDS, *Social Science and Medicine*, 38: 1347–65.

Crawford, R. (2006) Health as a meaningful social practice, *Health*, 10(4): 401–20.

Crewe, M. and Aggleton, P. (2003) Racism, HIV/AIDS and Africa: some issues revisited, *South African Journal of International Affairs*, 10: 139–49.

Davies, M. (1997) Shattered assumptions: time and the experience of long-term HIV positivity, *Social Science and Medicine*, 44(5): 561–71.

Dyer, S.J., Abrahams, N., Hoffman, M. and van der Spuy, Z.M. (2002) 'Men leave me as I cannot have children': women's experiences of involuntary childlessness, *Human Reproduction*, 17(6): 1663–8.

Ezzy, D. (2000) Illness narratives: time, hope and HIV, *Social Science and Medicine*, 50: 605–17.

Fagerlind, H., Ring, L., Brülde, B., Feltelius, N. and Lindblad, A.K. (2010) Patients' understanding of the concepts of health and quality of life, *Patient Education and Counselling*, 78: 104–10.

Foucault, M. (1977) *Discipline and Punish: The Birth of the Prison*. New York: Vintage.

Foucault, M. (1980) *Power/Knowledge: Selected Interviews and Other Writings, 1972–1977*. New York: Pantheon.

Foucault, M. (1984) Truth and power, in P. Rabinow (ed.) *The Foucault Reader: An Introduction to Foucault's Thoughts*. London: Penguin.

Foucault, M. (2004) *Anthologie*. Paris: Gallimard.

Garcia, K. K. (2007) The fat fight: the risks and consequences of the Federal Government's failing public health campaign, *Faculty Scholarship Series*, Paper #11. Available at: http://digitalcommons.law.yale.edu/fss_papers/11 [accessed 18 October 2012].

Gergen, K.J. (1999) *An Invitation to Social Construction*. London: Sage.

Graham, H. (1987) Women's smoking and family health, *Social Science and Medicine*, 25(1): 47–56.

Hare-Mustin, R. and Marecek, J. (1997) Abnormal and clinical psychology: the politics of madness, in D. Fox and I. Prilleltensky (eds.) *Critical Psychology: An Introduction*. London: Sage.

Holland, J., Ramazanoglu, C. and Scott, S. (1990a) Managing risk and experiencing danger: tensions between government AIDS policy and young women's sexuality, *Gender and Education*, 2(2): 193–202.

Holland, J., Ramazanoglu, C., Scott, S., Sharp, S. and Thompson, R. (1990b) *Don't die of ignorance: I nearly died of embarrassment*, Paper presented to the Fourth Social Aspects of AIDS Conference, London.

Holland, J., Ramazanoglu, C., Scott, S., Sharpe, S. and Thomson, R. (1990c) Sex, gender and power: young women's sexuality in the shadow of AIDS, *Sociology of Health and Illness*, 12: 336–50.

Jacobus, M., Fox Keller, E. and Shuttleworth, S. (1990) *Body/Politics: Women and the Discourses of Science*. London: Routledge.

Jordanova, L. (1995) The social construction of medical knowledge, *Social History of Medicine*, 8(3): 361–81.

Karp, D.A. (1996) *Speaking of Sadness: Depression, Disconnection and the Meaning of Illness*. New York: Oxford University Press.

Klitzman, R. and Beyer, R. (2003) *Mortal Secrets: Truth and Lies in the Age of AIDS*. Baltimore, MD: Johns Hopkins University Press.

Krieger, N. (2000) Refiguring 'race': epidemiology, racialized biology, and biological expressions of race relations, *International Journal of Health Services*, 30(1): 211–16.

Lupton, D. (1997) Foucault and the medicalisation critique, in R. Bunton and A. Petersen (eds.) *Foucault, Health and Medicine*. London: Routledge.

Lupton, D. (2000) The social construction of medicine and the body, in G.L. Albrecht, R. Fitzpatrick and S.C. Scrimshaw (eds.) *The Handbook of Social Studies in Health and Medicine*. London: Sage.

Myer, L. and Morroni, C. (2005) Supporting the sexual and reproductive rights of HIV-infected individuals, *South African Medical Journal*, 95: 852–3.

Nettleton, S. and Bunton, R. (1995) Sociological critiques of health promotion, in R. Bunton, S. Nettleton and R. Burrows (eds.) *The Sociology of Health Promotion: Critical Analysis of Lifestyle Consumption and Risk*. London: Routledge.

Pearson, M. (1986) Racist notions of ethnicity and health, in S. Rodmell and A. Watt (eds.) *The Politics of Health Education*. London: Routledge & Kegan Paul.

Peyrot, M., McMurry, J.F. and Hedges, R. (1987) Living with diabetes, in J.A. Roth and P. Conrad (eds.) *The Experience and Management of Chronic Illness*. Greenwich, CT: JAI Press.

Sabatier, R. (1988) *Blaming Others: Prejudice, Race and Worldwide AIDS*. Washington, DC: Panos Institute.

Schneider, J.W. and Conrad, P. (1983) *Having Epilepsy: The Experience and Control of Illness*. Philadelphia, PA: Temple University Press.

Schulze, B. and Angermeyer, M.C. (2003) Subjective experiences of stigma: a focus group study of schizophrenic patients, their relatives and mental health professionals, *Social Science and Medicine*, 56: 299–312.

Shefer, T. and Foster, D. (2001) Discourses on women's (hetero)sexuality and desire in a South African local context, *Culture, Health and Sexuality*, 3: 375–90.

Sheiham, H. and Quick, A. (1982) *The Rickets Report*. London: Haringey CHC and CRC.

Shoveller, J.A., Johnson, J.L., Langillec, D.B. and Mitchell, T. (2004) Socio-cultural influences on young people's sexual development, *Social Science and Medicine*, 59: 473–87.

Smith, G., Bartlett, A. and King, M. (2004) Treatments of homosexuality in Britain since the 1950s – an oral history: the experience of patients, *British Medical Journal*, 328(7437): 427–9.

Stillwaggon, E. (2003) Racial metaphors: interpreting sex and AIDS in Africa, *Development and Change*, 34(5): 809–32.

Thorogood, N. (1992) Sex education as social control, *Critical Public Health*, 3(2): 43–50.

Thorogood, N. (1995) 'London dentist in HIV scare': HIV and dentistry in popular discourse, in R. Bunton, S. Nettleton and R. Burrow (eds.) *The Sociology of Health Promotion: Critical Analysis of Lifestyle Consumption and Risk*. London: Routledge.

Treichler, P.A. (1989) AIDS, homophobia, and biomedical discourse: an epidemic of signification, in D. Crimp (ed.) *AIDS: Cultural Analysis, Cultural Activism*. Cambridge, MA: MIT Press.

Turner, B.S. (1995) *Medical Power and Social Knowledge* (2nd edn.). Thousand Oaks, CA: Sage.

Ussher, J.M. (1991) *Women's Madness: Misogyny or Mental Illness?*. New York: Harvester Wheatsheaf.

Ussher, J.M. (1996) Premenstrual syndrome: reconciling disciplinary divides through the adoption of a material-discursive epistemological standpoint, *Annual Review of Sex Research*, 7: 218–51.

Watney, S. (1989) The spectacle of AIDS, in D. Crimp (ed.) *AIDS: Cultural Analysis, Cultural Activism*. Cambridge, MA: MIT Press.

Wilbraham, L. (2004) Discursive practice: analysing a Lovelines text on sex communication for parents, in D. Hook (ed.) *Critical Psychology*. Cape Town: UCT Press.

Williams, D.R., Lavizzo-Mourey, R. and Warren, R.C. (1994) The concept of race and health status in America, *Public Health Reports*, 109(1): 25–41.

Wilton, T. (1997) *EnGendering AIDS: Deconstructing Sex, Text and Epidemic*. London: Sage.

Wilton, T. and Aggleton, P. (1990) *Condoms, coercion and control: heterosexuality and the limits to HIV/AIDS education*, Paper presented to the Fourth Social Aspects of AIDS Conference, London.

Wood, C. and Foster, D. (1995) 'Being the type of lover …': gender-differentiated reasons for non-use of condoms by sexually active heterosexual students, *Psychology in Society*, 20: 13–35.

Further reading

Bunton, R. and Petersen, A. (eds.) (1997) *Foucault, Health and Medicine*. London: Routledge.

Bunton, R., Nettleton, S. and Burrows, R. (eds.) (1995) *The Sociology of Health Promotion* (Part II: Socio-political Critiques of Health Promotion). London: Routledge.

Burr, V. (1995) *An Introduction to Social Construction*. London: Routledge.

Chandler, D. (2008) *Semiotics for Beginners*. Available at: http://www.aber.ac.uk/media/Documents/S4B/sem06.html.

Conrad, P. and Barker, K.K. (2010) The social construction of illness: key insights and policy implications, *Journal of Health and Social Behavior*, 51: 67–79.

Evans, J. and Hall, S. (1999) Introduction, in J. Evans and S. Hall (eds.) *Visual Culture: The Reader*. London: Sage.

Hall, S. (1997) The work of representation, in S. Hall (ed.) *Representation: Cultural Representations and Signifying Practices*. London: Sage in association with the Open University (in particular pp. 13–39).

Lorber, J. (1997) *Gender and the Social Construction of Illness*. Thousand Oaks, CA: Sage.

Nikolas, R. (2006) *Politics of Life Itself: Biomedicine, Power and Subjectivity in the Twenty-First Century*. Princeton, NJ: Princeton University Press.

Roth, J.A. and Conrad, P. (eds.) (1987) *The Experience and Management of Chronic Illness*. Greenwich, CT: JAI Press.

Turner, B.S. (1995) *Medical Power and Social Knowledge* (2nd edn.). Thousand Oaks, CA: Sage.

What drives health promotion? 3

Wendy Macdowall, Ford Hickson, and Mark Petticrew

Overview

This chapter explores two questions. First, why are some health issues prioritized over others? Second, how are policy responses to those issues formulated? In doing so, the chapter discusses the complex processes that determine which needs health promotion seeks to address, whose needs it prioritizes, and what form it takes. It pays particular attention to how values, theory, and evidence influence the process of setting priorities for health promotion.

Learning objectives

After reading this chapter, you will be able to:

- identify factors important to the processes of policy formation in health promotion
- compare the challenges and opportunities presented by the evidence-based movement in public health and health promotion
- think critically about the nature of evidence and how it is generated, disseminated, interpreted and used

Key terms

Evidence: The available body of facts or information indicating whether a belief or proposition is true or valid (*Oxford English Dictionary*).

Evidence-based medicine: The conscientious, explicit, and judicious use of current best evidence in making decisions about the care of individual patients (Sackett et al., 1996).

Evidence-based public health: The conscientious, explicit and judicious use of current best evidence in making decisions about the care of communities and populations in the domain of health protection, disease prevention, health maintenance and improvement (Jenicek, 1997).

Policy: A course or principle of action adopted or proposed by an organization or individual (*Oxford English Dictionary*).

Policy agenda: The list of subjects or problems to which government officials and those close to them are paying serious attention to (Kingdon, 2002: 98).

Introduction

In the promotion of health and well-being, there are many different issues that governments could attend to. This begs the questions why, and how, are some issues acted on and others not, and why, and how, are some issues prioritized over others? A simple way of conceptualizing these questions is to consider two axes, one of need and one of action (see Figure 3.1). All other things being equal, we could reasonably expect that governments are more likely to take action as more need is identified. We might also expect the reverse to hold true – where there is little evidence of need (or evidence of little need), the likelihood of government action to meet that need is low. In many instances, this is indeed the case. For example, in 2011 the Department of Health in England set out its commitment to address obesity as a leading cause of diabetes, coronary heart disease, and cancer, which contribute significantly to the overall burden of disease and health care costs (Department of Health, 2011). However, there are numerous situations where government inaction occurs in the face of relatively high need and where government action occurs despite relatively low need. For example, during the 1990s and early 2000s, the Government of South Africa was widely criticized for not acting to address the growing crisis of HIV in the country.

It is therefore clear that simple evidence of the burden of disease does not automatically translate into public health actions. The reasons for this are varied and com-

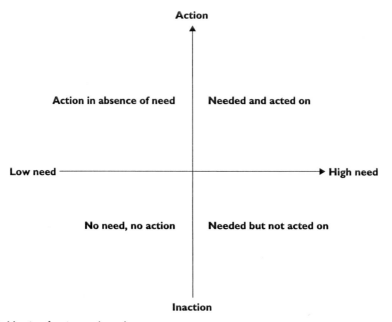

Figure 3.1 Matrix of action and need

plex and include issues related to: (1) how the causes of the 'need' are understood; (2) how those 'in need' are perceived; (3) how addressing the 'need' is conceptualized; and (4) interpretations of the evidence base and its shortfalls. In exploring these issues, definitions are important: How is need defined? Is a high level of disease sufficient evidence of need for action? Whose needs are these? Whose needs are more important? Who gets to decide these questions? There are political and ethical dimensions to all these questions. Also important is how the often competing interests of different actors – who may also have their own strongly held political and ethical values – are resolved. The political and ethical aspects of health promotion are considered in more detail in Chapter 4 of this book.

The policy process

To understand why some health issues are prioritized over others and how responses to those issues are formulated, is to understand how policy is made, adopted and implemented, and the factors that influence it. The policy development process is not always smooth and rational. In fact, public policy-making has been described as 'extraordinarily messy' (Kingdon, 2002: 97). Kingdon goes on to argue that it does have 'a sort of structure, but there is plenty of room for complexity, uncertainty, fluidity and residual randomness' (p. 97).

A number of different frameworks and models have been developed to analyse and/ or describe policy-making. Walt (1994) introduces the health policy triangle to help us think systematically about the different factors that may affect policy. It focuses on the three dimensions of content (of policy), context (within which policy-making occurs), and process (of policy-making). Within the triangle are the actors involved (individuals, groups, organizations).

A common framework for policy-making distinguishes four distinct stages, each with its own set of questions (see Box 3.1).

Box 3.1 Stages in the policy process

Stage 1: Problem identification and issue recognition
How do issues get on to the policy agenda? Why are some issues not even discussed?

Stage 2: Policy formation
Who formulates policy? How is it formulated? Where do initiatives come from?

Stage 3: Policy implementation
Who must act differently? What resources are available? Who should be involved? How can implementation be enforced?

Stage 4: Policy evaluation
What happens once a policy is put into effect? Is it monitored? Does it achieve its objectives? Does it have unintended consequences? Is it sustained or abandoned?

Source: Adapted from Walt (1994).

This framework can be both descriptive (it is what happens) and prescriptive (it is what should happen). In practice, how far these stages are followed in a logical, sequential set of steps is a matter of debate. It is also worth noting that models usually present the policy process as linear, while in practice policies may get stuck at any one stage in the process or may be sidelined or abandoned. Models of the policy process should, therefore, always be seen as idealized versions of reality.

There are three main models that address rational policy-making: the rational, incremental, and mixed scanning. The *rational model*, as the name suggests, proposes that having identified a problem, policy-makers (do or should) systematically gather and assess a variety of policy options and their potential outcomes, and having done so select the one that is most likely to address their goals. However, there are many factors that constrain policy-makers from behaving rationally. Walt (1994) identified four main factors: (1) the challenge of problem definition as it may not always be clear what the specific problem is; (2) the challenge of weighing up alternative policy options in the absence of definitive information; (3) the fact that policy-makers themselves are not objective, as their own values will influence how they conceptualize both the problems and the potential solutions; and (4) that previous policies will influence and potentially limit current policy options. Together these factors mean that some areas of known need are not acted on, and sometimes actions are taken when there is little or no evidence of need.

An alternative to the rational model of policy process is that of *incrementalism*. According to Lindblom (1959), the constraints on policy-makers preclude them from assessing all of the evidence and considering the full range of policy options. In practice, they consider only a limited number of alternatives that do not radically differ from the *status quo*. He describes the process as muddling through and of being influenced by partisan mutual adjustment (the positioning and repositioning of various interested parties). As such, Lindblom argues that what is possible politically is most commonly only incrementally different from what went before. For policy to progress, policy-makers must agree on a direction of travel. Where all actors disagree, or where there are two powerful but opposing sides, policy gets 'stuck' and it becomes impossible to move forward. From this perspective, the measure of a good decision is the extent to which decision-makers agree about it. This model of policy-making has its own problems. Where the rational model is criticized for being too idealistic, the incremental model is criticized for its conservatism. It is argued that within this model it is not possible to make the step changes that are often required for significant health gain.

Recognizing the idealism of the rational approach and the conservativism of the incrementalist approach, a middle position, that of *mixed scanning*, has been proposed by Etzioni (1967). The term scanning refers to an array of activities carried out to aid decision-making, including searching for, collating, and evaluating information. In mixed scanning, decisions are classified into two levels, namely fundamental (macro) decisions and small (micro) decisions. The model proposes that good policy decision-making uses different degrees of scanning for different levels, and that not all decisions require the same exhaustive assessment of the evidence. Some macro decisions can be taken without the micro-detail of all the implications of that decision being known.

Policy agenda-setting

Kingdon (2002) proposes that there are three streams to policy-making that occur simultaneously and in tandem: problems, proposals, and politics. This is a way of conceptualizing the processes at play in limiting the list to those issues that actually are the focus of attention, known as policy agenda-setting. He describes how the three streams flow around governments largely independently of each other (see Box 3.2). He argues that 'proposals are generated whether or not policy makers are solving a problem, problems are recognised whether or not there is a solution and political events move along according to their own dynamic' (Kingdon, 2002: 98). He goes on to argue that there are critical times of opportunity when the three streams align to open a 'policy window'. So-called policy entrepreneurs can exploit the opening of a policy window to push their issue or their solution.

Box 3.2 Kingdon's agenda-setting streams

Problem stream: where issues are identified and problematized. It has both objective and subjective elements. Objectively, changes in indicators of various health behaviours and health outcomes can draw attention to certain issues. As can certain 'focussing events', such as a scientific breakthrough that attracts media attention. However, there is also a more subjective process of interpretation that renders something as a 'problem' that we feel we ought to do something about. This interpretation is influenced by how issues are framed and whether they conflict with prevailing values.

Proposal stream: where policy proposals are created and honed. Many actors, including civil servants, politicians, researchers, interest groups, activists, and policy analysts, all contribute ideas that have policy potential. It is argued that how ideas are selected is analogous to the primordial soup: 'Ideas, like molecules, bump into one another, combining and recombining in various ways ... In the process of policy evolution some ideas fall away, others survive and prosper, and some are selected to become serious contenders for adoption' (p. 101).

Political stream: where features of the political environment influence the policy agenda, such as changes in governments, shifts in public opinion and interest group pressure.

Source: Adapted from Kingdon (2002).

Activity 3.1

Identify a health issue that has come to prominence in your country recently. Using Kingdon's (2002) agenda-setting model, can you identify factors from the problem, proposal, and political streams that influenced why the issue came onto the agenda or rose up it?

Feedback

In the problem stream you may have identified the publication of regional, national or international health statistics or indicators, or the publication of a major piece of research. Or maybe there was a crisis (for example, an outbreak of a disease). In the policy stream you may have identified the publication of an influential report or guidance offering policy options or some activity by key politicians or civil servants (for example, a high-profile conference). In the political stream you may have identified a change in government, a change in public opinion around the issues or actions of interest groups or of individual champions. Kingdon argues that issues are only taken seriously by governments when the three streams come together.

Hall et al. (1975) have proposed an alternative model of policy agenda-setting. This model suggests that an issue will only receive attention when it has high levels of legitimacy, feasibility, and support. *Legitimacy* refers to those issues that the government feel that they should be concerned with, or have the right to intervene on. These vary considerably between countries and within counties. There are many issues where the boundaries of what it is acceptable for the state to intervene on – and the nature of any intervention – are fiercely contested. For example, the extent to which the state should act on the economy varies enormously across different countries. Some people believe the state has little or no role in the economy (for example, free marketeers), whereas others think the state should strongly intervene on issues such as interest rates, banking, and monopolies. Other areas where the state's role is strongly contested include family life, religion, education, the media, and health. *Feasibility* refers to the extent to which government feels it has the ability and resources to address the issue. Finally, *support* refers to public support for intervention. Although some types of political regimes are less dependent on public support, such as dictatorships, even in these regimes there is a need for support for policy among key groups, such as the armed forces (Buse et al., 2012).

The importance of public support

A difficult issue for any government in relation to health promotion policy, and central to the question of public support, is how far it is acceptable to intervene in people's lives to promote their own health, or that of others. Richard Reeves, in his 2010 report to the UK Government on the role of the state in health and well-being argues: 'Good health is a vital ingredient of a good life – but so is freedom' (Reeves, 2010: 4). He conducted qualitative research with members of the public and found that people are more likely to support action on policy issues where freedom of choice is protected and where there is a strong case for intervention because there is seen to be sound evidence to justify it. His research also highlighted the public's desire for government to act in helping make healthier choices easier by the regulation of industry. This suggests it is more palatable to the British public for industry to be regulated than have their own behaviour regulated. It may also indicate where the public see the responsibility lies for some health issues and highlights the role of industry as a key player in the policy process.

Even when health promotion policies are targeted at specific groups rather than seeking to reach the whole population, public support remains important. One of the factors that influences public support for more targeted interventions, and therefore the likelihood and nature of the intervention, is how the public perceive those affected. The policy response to HIV/AIDS is a case in point. Watney (1997) and others have argued that in the UK in the 1980s there was a limited public health response to cases of AIDS while it appeared confined to 'homosexuals and addicts'.

Reeves (2010) concludes that government should ask themselves three questions before intervening. The first relates to *legitimacy* and asks how strong is the case for intervention? The second relates to individual *autonomy* and asks how can the state respond in a way that protects (or increases) autonomy? The third relates to *effectiveness* and asks will it work? This summary may sound eminently sensible on the surface, but the concepts of legitimacy, autonomy, and effectiveness are all contested and value-laden. It is also of note that while in principle these questions may be transferable to other contexts, they have been constructed in the context of the UK. The ethical principle of autonomy is considered in Chapter 4 of this book. Here, we now turn to the role of evidence and in particular the concept of evidence-based decision-making, which are key to questions of legitimacy and of effectiveness.

The role of evidence

The evidence-based movement began in the field of medicine in the early 1990s. At its core is the principle that clinical decisions should be made 'on the basis of the best available scientific data, rather than on customary practices or the personal beliefs of the health care provider' (Des Jarlais et al., 2004: 361). Evidence-based medicine also recognizes that many health care decisions have been made simply out of convenience or they in some way were beneficial to the provider (for example, they were less costly). The concept of evidence-based medicine has gained currency since its inception and there are now similar movements in public health, health promotion, and many other fields of public policy. This proliferation of the concept is rooted in the view that, like health professionals, those involved in policy initiatives or programme management should also base their decisions on the best available scientific information. This raises questions, however, about the nature of evidence, including: What counts as 'evidence'? What is the 'best' evidence? This in turn raises questions about the research that underpins that evidence: How is the research funded and by whom? How is it generated and by whom? How is it interpreted and by whom? How is it used and by whom?

Activity 3.2

What different types of evidence can help inform decision-making in health promotion policy and practice? Remember that evidence consist of facts or information that supports or refutes a belief.

Feedback

It is likely that you thought about how evidence can help both identify problems and their causes and suggest how best to address them. Brownson et al. (2009) suggests three types of evidence. The first type of evidence indicates that 'something should be done' (it defines the causes of disease and the size and strength of preventable risk); the second type indicates that 'specifically this intervention should be done' (it describes the relative effectiveness of different interventions); and the third type indicates 'how something should be done' (it informs the implementation of interventions). There is more of the first type of evidence and less of the second and third types (Brownson et al., 2009). This means we know about more problems than solutions.

Types of evidence (or hierarchies of evidence)

Since the establishment of evidence-based medicine, there has been considerable debate about what constitutes 'evidence' and what the 'best' evidence is. Parallel debates have taken place in relation to evidence-based public health and health promotion. Figure 3.2 provides an example of a suggested hierarchy based on the relative objectivity of different types of evidence. In evidence-based medicine, randomized control trials sit at the top of the hierarchy of research study designs for assessing effectiveness, with systematic reviews of randomized controlled trials considered to be the strongest form of evidence of effectiveness. A number of distinctions have been made between evidence-based medicine and evidence-based public health and health promotion, and one of the questions that has been hotly debated is whether the evidence-based medicine 'model' – which prizes randomized controlled trials and systematic reviews – 'fits' the world of social interventions. It has been argued that reluctance to apply evidence-based medicine principles to public health and health promotion is based on a number of misconceptions and misunderstandings (Macintyre and Petticrew, 2000).

Tannahill (2008) identifies three issues that are particular to evidence of effectiveness in health promotion. These are demand, skewing, and inadequacy. In relation to the demand for effectiveness evidence, Tannahill argues that there are so many health topics (e.g. cardiovascular disease, cancer, obesity, sexual health, and mental health), behavioural topics (e.g. smoking, diet, alcohol consumption, and physical activity), life stages (e.g. preconception, pregnancy, early years, adolescence, middle age, and late life), settings (e.g. schools, workplaces, social care), and cross-cutting themes (e.g. the social determinants and inequalities in health), combined with different levels of action (e.g. individual, community, and environment), that there will never be evidence of effectiveness on all potential interventions. In relation to skewing of effectiveness evidence, Tannahill suggests that 'the conventional approach [derived from evidence based medicine] has left a legacy of skewing the search for, and supply of, effectiveness evidence towards interventions relating to specific health or risk factor topics and on the "inner layers" of the health improvement onion' (Tannahill, 2008: 382). In relation to inadequacy of effectiveness evidence, he argues that the 'actions and types of action for which evidence is strongest are not necessarily the most important for achieving population health gain and reducing health inequalities' (ibid.). In summary, the best

- Scientific literature in systematic reviews
- Scientific literature in one or more journal articles
- Public health surveillance data
- Programme evaluations
- Qualitative data
  - Community members
  - Other stakeholders
- Media/marketing data
- Word of mouth
- Personal experience

Objective

Subjective

Figure 3.2 Different forms of public health evidence
Source: Brownson et al. (2009)

evidence we have is about the simplest interventions. We have less – or weaker – evidence about complex interventions (such as policies) but policy-makers are often most interested in complex questions. This has also been called the 'inverse evidence law' (Nutbeam, 2004).

In addition to questions about effectiveness, there is growing recognition of the need to consider questions of context. These questions include how interventions work, why they work, and for whom they work. In 2011, Waters and colleagues detailed the essential components of public health and health promotion evidence reviews. The authors argue that 'if reviews of intervention evidence are to be useful to decision-makers at all, contextual and implementation information is an essential, non-negotiable component of the review process' (Waters et al., 2011: 462). They go on to make a number of recommendations to ensure public health and health promotion evidence reviews are useful to decision-makers, including: engaging stakeholders when scoping the review; understanding the pathways in operation and the theoretical underpinnings of the evidence; and capturing information on programme implementation through the review process (Waters et al., 2011).

Use of evidence by policy-makers

In practice, how research findings are used and what using research to inform policy and practice actually means vary considerably (Weiss, 1979). Different models of research utilization acknowledge that the linear interpretation of knowledge-driven use, which goes from basic research through applied research to application, rarely occurs in reality. A more commonly applied model, which is also linear, is the problem-solving or knowledge-deficit model where a problem exists, or a commitment to 'do some-thing' has been made, but information regarding the solution is lacking and is actively sought. Two other models, which appear to reflect the often messy, non-linear process of policy-making described above, are the interactive and the enlightenment models. The interactive model acknowledges that there are many pieces in the policy jigsaw and that research is only one part. The enlightenment model suggests that in practice research 'diffuses circuitously though manifold channels' (Weiss, 1979: 429) and over time enters the policy sphere. It is argued, however, that this non-direct mechanism renders research findings susceptible to both oversimplification and to distortion (Weiss, 1979). Evidence is also used – and abused – in other ways. It may be used to meet political ends, where research findings are picked selectively and used to support a decision already made, which Weiss (1979) describes thus: 'research as ammunition'. It may also be used tactically, for example to pass on responsibility for unpopular policy.

Whether or not research is used for purely political purposes, it is important to acknowledge the central role of politics in any understanding of the research–policy interface. In the first instance, decisions regarding what research gets funded may be made for political reasons rather than for scientific ones. Furthermore, whether research findings are acted upon and result in any changes to policy and practice is essentially the domain of politics. As Oliver (2006: 195) puts it, 'Science can identify solutions to pressing public health problems, but only politics can turn most of those solutions into reality.' That is not to say that the process cannot be influenced by the academics or others who generate the research or by other actors in the policy proc-ess, but it is to say that this is an inherently political enterprise.

Research conducted with policy-makers to explore how evidence informs public health policy-making has highlighted some common themes that militate against research informing policy (Petticrew et al., 2004; Rychetnick and Wise, 2004). These include:

- Researchers lacking an understanding of the practical and political constraints on policy-makers.
- Policy-makers having a more pluralistic view of evidence than the narrowly defined research-based findings.
- Researchers failing to make the practical and policy implications of their findings explicit.

Rychetnick and Wise (2004) suggest that academics may be reluctant to express their views on the implications of their findings, let alone get involved in publicly advocating for particular policies for a number of reasons. They speculate that this reserve may be linked to the scientific convention of sticking to the demonstrated facts. They may have concerns regarding the imperative to remain impartial. They may lack knowledge about the policy process and how to influence it. It is also the case that evidence given by disinterested parties is often viewed as more valid than that presented by someone who is clearly already committed to a particular course of action.

Nutley and colleagues (2002) identify a number of key requirements if evidence is to have a greater impact on policy and practice (see Box 3.3).

Box 3.3 Key requirements if evidence is to have a greater impact on policy and practice

1 Agreement as to what counts as evidence in what circumstances.
2 A strategic approach to the creation of evidence in priority areas, with concomitant systematic efforts to accumulate evidence in the form of robust bodies of knowledge.
3 Effective dissemination of evidence to where it is most needed and the development of effective means of providing wide access to knowledge.
4 Initiatives to ensure the integration of evidence into policy and encourage the utilization of evidence in practice.

Source: Nutley et al. (2002).

Social research ideas also work their way into policy through featuring in popular publications and the general media. Policy-makers are attuned to the current zeitgeist and respond accordingly. There are trends and fads in policy-making as much as there are in fashion and music. Popular books for a general readership are much more likely to be the source of new inspiration in health policy-making than are specialist papers in academic journals. Some examples of popular big idea books in the health arena include: *The Tipping Point: How Little Things Can Make a Big Difference* by Malcolm Gladwell, first published in 2000; *The Wisdom of Crowds: Why the Many are Smarter than the Few and How Collective Wisdom Shapes Business, Economies, Societies and Nations* by James Surowiecki, published in 2004; *The Status Syndrome: How Your Social Standing Directly Affects Your Health and Life Expectancy* by Michael Marmot, published in 2004; and *Nudge: Improving Decisions about Health, Wealth, and Happiness* by Richard H. Thaler and Cass R. Sunstein, published in 2008. These books have made a significant, but sometimes short-term, impact on health policy-makers, illustrating the fact that knowledge alone is not sufficient to influence policy. Knowledge must also be packaged and promoted for it to have an effect.

So to influence policy, research findings need to be clearly presented, timely, and relevant to current debates. They should be made available in a non-technical language that policy-makers can understand and then disseminated through channels they will encounter or can easily access. Although evidence of effectiveness may not change, or may change very slowly, evidence of unmet health need should be as up-to-date as possible if it is to be used to inform health-promoting action. Systems also need to be in place for relevant scientific information to be identified, synthesized, and disseminated. In many parts of the world, these systems are not well developed (Petticrew et al., 2004).

Tannahill (2008) argues that we should think of evidence-*informed* health promotion rather than evidence-*based* health promotion. This chimes with Nutley and colleagues' (2002: 1) view that 'evidence based' when attached as a modifier to policy or practice 'can obscure the sometimes limited role that evidence can, does, or even should, play'.

Activity 3.3

Reflect on what you have learnt about the role of evidence in developing health promotion policy. What do you think are the potential advantages of an evidence-informed approach in health promotion? What do you think are the potential limitations of such an approach?

Feedback

You might have reflected that the advantages of an evidence-informed approach could include:

- Greater consensus on the rationale for intervention
- Greater support for intervention
- A greater chance of achieving the desired outcomes by employing strategies that have been demonstrated to work
- A more judicious use of resources
- Increased understanding of areas where more research is needed.

You might have reflected on limitations, including:

- Innovative approaches may not get adopted as there is no evidence to support them
- Problems for which no clear solutions have been shown to be effective may get sidelined
- Evidence is not always taken up and is sometimes used inappropriately or out of context
- Evidence that is perceived as more subjective, for example how well people feel themselves to be, may be undermined
- Decisions about funding research may be politically driven
- Evidence cannot compensate for a lack of political will to deal with a problem.

What about theory?

In much of the debate about evidence-based policy and practice, the role of theory has received relatively little attention (Green, 2000). At first sight it may seem that there is a contradiction in using evidence to inform policy and practice and in using theory. It may even be tempting to assume that evidence can replace theory in developing and implementing health promotion initiatives. However, as this book makes clear, theory is essential to how health 'problems' and their causes are understood and throughout the processes of developing, implementing, and evaluating solutions to those 'problems'. Theory is also crucial in informing policy and practice in the many areas where gaps exist in the evidence base. Furthermore, evidence is derived from the testing of theory, whether explicitly stated or not (Tannahill, 2008).

A framework for health promotion policy and practice decision-making

The framework shown in Figure 3.3 encapsulates the important dimensions of health promotion decision-making that have been introduced in this chapter. This model draws on Walt's (1994) health policy triangle and the health policy decision-making framework for health promotion proposed by Tannahill (2008). It considers the role of evidence *and* theory, ethics *and* politics, and the processes and actors involved. Inherent in all of these dimensions are values, which are at the centre of the proposed model. All of the elements in the model influence how health need is understood, prioritized, and translated into health promotion policy and then practice.

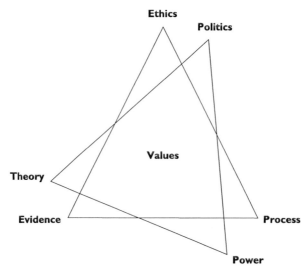

Figure 3.3 A framework for health promotion policy and practice decision-making

Summary

This chapter has explored factors that influence how health need is understood, prioritized, and translated into health promotion policy and then practice. It has shown that the policy process is complex and often messy. While theoretical models are useful in helping to understand this process, they often reflect an idealized version of reality. This chapter has also described how the concept of evidence-based policy and practice has gained currency in health promotion and other areas of public policy in recent years and introduced the debate about what counts as 'evidence' and what is the 'best' evidence. It has explained many factors that influence how policy-makers use evidence. Finally, the chapter proposes that evidence, theory, ethics, politics, and values interact in complex ways to drive the promotion of health.

References

Brownson, R.C., Fielding, J.E. and Maylahn, C.M. (2009) Evidence-based public health: a fundamental concept for public health practice, *Annual Review of Public Health*, 30: 175–201.

Buse, K., Mays, N. and Walt, G. (2012) *Making Health Policy*. Maidenhead: Open University Press.

Department of Health (2011) *Healthy Lives, Healthy People: A Call to Action on Obesity in England*. London: Department of Health.

Des Jarlais, D.C., Lyles, C., Crepaz, N. and the TREND Group (2004) Improving the reporting quality of nonrandomized evaluations of behavioral and public health interventions: the TREND statement, *American Journal of Public Health*, 94(3): 361–6.

Etzioni, A. (1967) Mixed-scanning: a 'third' approach to decision-making, *Public Administration Review*, 27(5): 385–92.

Gladwell, M. (2000) *The Tipping Point: How Little Things Can Make a Big Difference*. Boston, MA: Little, Brown & Co.

Green, J. (2000) The role of theory in evidence-based health promotion practice, *Health Education Research*, 15(2): 125–9.

Hall, P., Land, H., Parker, R. and Webb, A. (1975) *Change, Choice and Conflict in Social Policy*. London: Heinemann.

Jenicek, M. (1997) Epidemiology, evidenced-based medicine, and evidence-based public health, *Journal of Epidemiology*, 7: 187–97 (erratum, *Journal of Epidemiology*, 8: 76; 1998).

Kingdon, J.W. (2002) The reality of public policy making, in M. Danis, C. Clancy and L.R. Churchill (eds.) *Ethical Dimensions of Health Policy*. Oxford: Oxford University Press.

Lindblom, C.E. (1959) The science of 'muddling through', *Public Administration Review*, 19(2): 79–88.

Macintyre, S. and Petticrew, P. (2000) Good intentions and received wisdom are not enough, *Journal of Epidemiology and Community Health*, 54: 802–3.

Marmot, M. (2004) *The Status Syndrome: How Your Social Standing Directly Affects Your Health and Life Expectancy*. New York: Owl Books.

Nutbeam, D. (2004) Getting evidence into policy and practice to address health inequalities, *Health Promotion International*, 19(2): 137–40.

Nutley, S., Davies, H. and Walter, I. (2002) *Evidence based policy and practice: cross sector lessons from the UK*. Working Paper #20. St. Andrews: ESRC UK Centre for Evidence Based Policy and Practice, Research Unit for Research Utilisation.

Oliver, T.R. (2006) The politics of public health policy, *Annual Review of Public Health*, 27: 195–233.

Petticrew, M., Whitehead, M., Macintyre, S.J., Graham, H. and Egan, M. (2004) Evidence for public health policy on inequalities: 1: The reality according to policymakers, *Journal of Epidemiology and Community Health*, 58: 811–16.

Reeves, R.A. (2010) *Liberal Dose? The Role of the State in Health and Well Being*. London: Department of Health. Available at: http://www.dh.gov.uk/prod_consum_dh/groups/dh_digitalassets/@dh/@en/@ps/documents/digitalasset/dh_111695.pdf [accessed 19 March 2013].

Rychetnik, L. and Wise, M. (2004) Advocating evidence-based health promotion: reflections and a way forward, *Health Promotion International*, 19(2): 247–57.

Sackett, D.L., Rosenberg, W.M.C., Muir Gray, J.A., Haynes, R.B. and Richardson, W.S. (1996) Evidence based medicine: what it is and what it isn't, *British Medical Journal*, 312(7023): 71–2.

Surowiecki, J. (2004) *The Wisdom of Crowds: Why the Many are Smarter than the Few and How Collective Wisdom Shapes Business, Economies, Societies and Nations*. New York: Random House.

Tannahill, A. (2008) Beyond evidence – to ethics: a decision-making framework for health promotion, public health and health improvement, *Health Promotion International*, 23(4): 380–90.

Thaler, R.H. and Sunstein, C.R. (2008) *Nudge: Improving Decisions about Health, Wealth, and Happiness*. New Haven, CT: Yale University Press.

Walt, G. (1994) *Health Policy: An Introduction to Process and Power*. London: Zed Books.

Waters, E., Hall, B., Armstrong, R., Doyle, J., Pettman, T. and de Silva-Sanigorski, A. (2011) Cochrane update: Essential components of public health evidence reviews: capturing intervention complexity, implementation, economics and equity, *Journal of Public Health*, 33(3): 462–5.

Watney, S. (1997) *Policing Desire: Pornography, AIDS and the Media* (3rd edn.). London: Cassell.

Weiss, C.H. (1979) The many meanings of research utilization, *Public Administration Review*, 39(5): 426–31.

Further reading

Buse, K., Mays, N. and Walt, G. (2012) *Making Health Policy*. Maidenhead: Open University Press.

Political and ethical considerations

4

Nick Fahy

Overview

You have already learnt that health promotion raises political and ethical issues that need to be taken into account for health promotion to be effective, and to be seen as acceptable. These include issues linked to the relationship between individuals and society, who has the right to decide and the basis on which health promotion is justified. Taking these as a starting point, this chapter will look at some theoretical approaches for considering such issues in political and ethical philosophy and how they are resolved in practice.

Learning objectives

After reading this chapter, you will be able to:

- describe some of the key political and ethical issues relevant to health promotion
- relate these issues to some alternative philosophical approaches and consider their usefulness in resolving health promotion questions
- consider how these political and ethical issues are addressed in practice

Key terms

Beneficence: Doing good; active kindness.

Liberalism: The rights of the individual should be respected to enable society as a whole to benefit from the full potential of all its citizens.

Neoliberalism: A modern variation on liberalism, typically used in the context of the role of the state, emphasizing market-based solutions to problems rather than public intervention.

Non-maleficence: A principle based on avoiding the causation of harm.

Plato's Republic: An ideal society governed by those best qualified to do so.

Utilitarianism: A theory of the good (whatever yields the greatest utility or value) and a theory of the right (the right act is that which yields the greatest net utility).

Introduction

There is much scope for political debate and dispute on the ends and means of health promotion. This is something that health professionals need to be aware of in their work. First, over the result to be attained, what is good health? This may appear a straightforward question but, as you have seen in Chapters 1, 2, and 3, people may have different understandings of what health means in practice. Examples include those linked to self-image (such as obesity and nutrition), behavioural choices (such as smoking, alcohol or drug-taking), sexual behaviour (linked to sexually transmitted diseases), or mental health (and attitudes towards depression or suicide). And where there are differences, this leads to the question about whose definition of health should take precedence – that of the health professional, the individual concerned, or society as a whole?

Second, there may also be differences over the means used for promoting or achieving health. Political questions will arise in particular for those cases where the health-related behaviour of one person has an impact on the health of another, such as with smoking, alcohol consumption (potentially linked to violence), and vaccination (where the benefit is also for the surrounding population). There is also the issue of the cost of treating avoidable ill health, and how far the solidarity of the community gives that community a right to impose their views on the individuals depending on that solidarity – such as making smokers contribute to the cost of their own care, or not funding certain types of medical intervention such as abortion.

Third, health is affected by factors such as unemployment, housing, access to essential services, education, and the environment, which are discussed in more detail in Chapter 5. Action to improve health will require political decisions in these areas and the balancing of different priorities against each other. For example, there may be economic or commercial costs to action to promote health.

Looking at these areas of potential conflict, it is clear that there must be some mechanism for resolving differences of view within society, as with other choices about the organization of the community as a whole and limits on the behaviour of individuals within it. This brings us to the political philosophy and organization of the society in which you live and work, as these political mechanisms and values will be what determines how such issues are resolved in practice. Questions related to health and behaviour are among the most sensitive questions of modern political life, and thus it is essential for health professionals to be aware of this wider context to their work.

Activity 4.1

In this activity, you will relate the issues and approaches discussed in this chapter to your own situation and apply the theories put forward in practice.

1 Identify some political and ethical issues related to your area of work or study in health promotion. How are these issues resolved in practice?
2 What political or ethical frameworks are used by you or by others in your area of work or study? Are they compatible?

Feedback

1 There are likely to be quite a wide range of potential issues, including those mentioned in the introduction to this chapter. However, their political or ethical dimension may not be immediately obvious; they may not necessarily be considered through formal political or ethical structures but may be presented in a wide variety of different ways, depending on their specific context. How issues are presented will affect how they are resolved in practice. People may frame issues in different ways (for example, as a matter of individual choice rather than as a health issue) depending on the outcome that they would prefer.

2 Many different political and ethical frameworks are mentioned in everyday life. These are not limited to explicit political ideologies. Economic systems (socialism, capitalism) may also be linked to certain political values (collective responsibility, individual liberty). Different societies may have established values on certain issues. One clear example is religion; different religious beliefs involve different ethical approaches and may also have an impact on what mechanisms the people concerned accept for resolving conflicts.

A perfect society?

Questions about resolving different values and priorities within society are fundamental and have, therefore, been considered from the earliest works of political philosophy. For the first approach to addressing these issues, you can go back to one of the earliest works of political philosophy – Plato's *The Republic*, written over 3000 years ago in Greece (Plato, 1989). This was a time of city-states, where different cities within the relatively small geographical area around the Aegean organized themselves individually and quite differently, with consequently much discussion about what the best means of organization was. *The Republic* sets out Plato's answer, a perfect society – the Republic – which is governed by those best qualified to do so: the Guardians.

Plato's argument is that where some activity can be done better by people with more expertise, the best approach is to choose someone who has the appropriate expertise, put them in charge, and do as they say. Therefore, the best way to ensure that society is run as well as possible is to select the most capable people, give them all appropriate training, and put them in charge; these people are the Guardians, and they direct the behaviour of everyone else.

This is the ultimate vision of society in which decisions are taken based on expertise and evidence. Government is seen as an activity based on knowledge that can be done well or badly, like any other profession. Plato therefore argues that you should logically prefer it to be done well, and thus give the power of decision-making to those best qualified to exercise it; you should have the same type of relationship to the Guardians as patients have with their doctor.

Giving power to a small minority on the basis of some expertise or ability does not leave much room for democracy. This is entirely intentional by Plato, who did not view democratic rule as a good thing but rather as encouraging factionalism and selfishness. This 'perfect society' may seem quite alien to us today, with its disregard for individual freedoms and exclusion of most members of society from government. Nevertheless, though the society that Plato describes is very different from modern societies, the questions he raises are still relevant today.

Particularly relevant for health promotion is the tension between taking decisions on the basis of expertise and taking decisions on the basis of the majority view of all citizens, regardless of their knowledge or expertise in the area. In Plato's time, there were major advances towards a more scientific and empirical understanding of the world. This was part of the context in which Plato considered that good government should be based on expertise, not just the majority view. Similarly today, we increasingly seek scientifically based explanations and remedies for the problems that confront us, and place great trust in those who have the expertise to analyse and recommend on a scientific basis. The power of the Guardians of Plato's Republic prompted the question 'who will guard the Guardians?', and the same question applies to the authority of health professionals and other experts today. After all, if expertise is the basis of authority, this leads to questions about the basis of this expertise – how we know what the correct analysis or action is.

Activity 4.2

This activity encourages you to apply the concepts articulated by Plato in a modern context, and to raise some related issues for health promotion.

1 What are the advantages and disadvantages of giving power to experts to decide? Give examples of areas outside health promotion of each approach.
2 How can the authority or expertise of experts be monitored or judged?

Feedback

1 Advantages of giving power to experts to decide are mostly focused around the *outcome*; someone with expert knowledge of a technical area should produce a better outcome than someone without that expertise, all other things being equal. However, there are limits to when this will be the case, which your examples of disadvantages should reflect. In particular, expertise is only useful when the issue for decision is one where technical knowledge is *relevant* – not the case for a conflict of values, for example. And the technical knowledge of the area should be *sufficient* to give a clear answer; where there is disagreement between experts or knowledge is limited, other approaches are required.

Also, decisions by experts may not be appropriate where the process of deciding is itself important – for example, where commitment is required from other people for the decision to be implemented. If people have not been able to choose for themselves or at least been part of a decision-making process that they perceive as fair, they will be less likely to feel committed to implementing a decision in practice. For example, most modern societies take democratic approval as being the ultimate political endorsement for decisions, not expert views. Therefore, your counter-examples to government by experts could be any area of decision by majority vote. However, there are some areas where decisions are left to experts. Having interest rates set by an independent central bank would be one example.

2 On monitoring the authority or expertise of experts, your answer might consider mechanisms such as making the basis for expert decisions open, so that others with

expertise can also analyse them. Your answer might also include mechanisms whereby experts regulate themselves and consider what standards are required of experts, and how these can be upheld, for example through professional associations.

Utilitarianism or consequence-based theory

Utilitarianism is a suggested theoretical framework for morality, law, and politics that accepts the principle of utility as the basis of ethics. Utilitarianism is both a theory of the good and a theory of the right. As a theory of the good, utilitarianism is welfarist – that is, the good is whatever yields the greatest utility (pleasure, satisfaction, or in reference to an objective list of values). As a theory of the right, utilitarianism is consequentialist – that is, the right act is that which yields the greatest net utility. The origins of this theory can be found in the writings of Jeremy Bentham and John Stuart Mill.

Utilitarians offer many examples from daily life to argue that we all engage in a utilitarian method of calculating what should be done by balancing goals and resources and considering the needs of everyone affected. The principle of utility is the ultimate standard for all utilitarians, although recently there has been argument as to whether this pertains to particular acts, in particular circumstances, or to general rules that determine which actions are right and which are wrong. *Rule* utilitarians consider the consequences of adopting rules, whereas *act* utilitarians disregard rules and justify their acts by appealing directly to the principle of utility. For the rule utilitarian, an act's conformity to a justified rule makes it right and the rule is in no case expendable, even when following it in that particular situation does not maximize utility. For the act utilitarian, moral rules may be useful as rough guidelines but are expendable if they do not promote utility.

Worthington Hooker was a prominent nineteenth-century doctor and rule utilitarian. He addressed the rule of telling the truth as follows:

> The good which may be done by deception in a *few* cases, is almost as nothing compared with the evil which it does in *many*, when the prospect of its doing good was just as promising as it was in those in which it succeeded. And when we add to this the evil which would result from a *general* adoption of a system of deception, the importance of strict adherence to the truth in our intercourse with the sick, even on the ground of expediency, becomes incalculably great.
>
> (cited in Beauchamp and Childress, 2009: 340; emphasis in the original)

Act utilitarians consider many of the moral questions raised by technological developments impossible to address in terms of traditional moral rules. This has many strengths, hence its popularity among ethicists working in health policy and practice. The requirement for objective assessment of the interests of all concerned and of impartial choice to maximize good outcomes for these are apparently desirable norms of policy-making. Utilitarianism is also beneficence-based, seeing morality in terms of promoting welfare.

The utilitarian approach has been criticized, however. Beauchamp and Childress (2009: 341–2) raise three arguments in particular. The first is about immoral preferences; what if there are outcomes that bring great satisfaction to some, but which we would regard as immoral – exploiting the ill health of factory workers for the satisfaction of cheaper products, for example? A second criticism is that utilitarianism seems to require us to act against our own interest if doing so would overall bring benefits. Thirdly, and perhaps most fundamentally, a utilitarian approach does not seem to protect the minority against the majority. In health promotion terms, if overall health could be promoted at the cost of the ill health of the few, the utilitarian approach would argue that it should be done, but would we accept that as ethical?

Liberalism and individual freedom

An alternative approach to resolving values and priorities in society is to focus not on the overall ideal outcome to be attained, as with Plato and the utilitarians, but on the rights of the individual. This 'liberal' approach of individual rights and the balance between the individual and society at large was articulated in particular by John Stuart Mill (1806–1873), and set out at the start of his essay *On Liberty*:

> The object of this Essay is to assert one very simple principle, as entitled to govern absolutely the dealings of society with the individual in the way of compulsion and control, whether the means used be physical force in the form of legal penalties or the moral coercion of public opinion. That principle is, that the sole end for which mankind are warranted, individually or collectively, in interfering with the liberty of action of any of their number, is self-protection. That the only purpose for which power can be rightfully exercised over any member of a civilised community, against his will, is to prevent harm to others. His own good, either physical or moral, is not a sufficient warrant. He cannot rightfully be compelled to do or forbear because it will make him happier, because, in the opinions of others, to do so would be wise, or even right. There are good reasons for remonstrating with him, or reasoning with him, or persuading him, or entreating him, but not for compelling him, or visiting him with any evil, in case he do otherwise. To justify that, the conduct from which it is desired to deter him must be calculated to produce evil to some one else. The only part of the conduct of any one, for which is amenable to society, is that which concerns others. In the part which merely concerns himself, his independence is, of right, absolute. Over himself, over his own body and mind, the individual is sovereign.
>
> (Mill, 1990: 135)

Mill argued that we should respect these freedoms of the individual both to enable them to realize their own potential and to enable society as a whole to benefit from the full potential of all its citizens. Mill only considers that this applies to adults 'in the maturity of their faculties'. For children, Mill considered that society has a specific responsibility to ensure proper education, to enable them to act rationally as adults and, if it fails, then society must bear the consequences. This liberal tradition was articulated alongside the revolutionary developments in industrialization and urbanization in Western Europe. As well as changes in economic structure, these times also brought major change in social organization, with greater individual freedom both economically and politically, and erosion of the established mechanisms for social control and standards. The liberal tradition gave a philosophical expression to these changes, and still forms a large part of the modern political framework of Western societies.

This philosophical approach sets a clear limit to the role of society in attempting to shape the behaviour of the individual – a limit that is especially applicable to health issues. Expertise or knowledge of the consequences of a particular kind of behaviour is no justification for interfering in a person's choices, on this basis. For example, the abuse of alcohol was one of the specific cases cited by Mill as something that might not be ideal behaviour but where society should not intervene unless it led to specific harm to someone else:

> No person ought to be punished simply for being drunk; but a soldier or a policeman should be punished for being drunk on duty. Whenever, in short, there is a definite damage, or a definite risk of damage, either to an individual or to the public, the case is taken out of the province of liberty, and is placed in that of morality or law.
>
> (Mill, 1990: 213)

Yet this also provides an example of the kind of argument that can be made against this liberal position. One might argue that in practical terms, for people living together in a society, the distinction between behaviour that causes harm to others and behaviour that is purely private is not as clear as Mill suggests – or at least, that the boundary of what does not affect others needs to be drawn much more narrowly than Mill describes. To continue the example of alcohol misuse, when someone drinks too much and causes harm to themselves, they also cause a burden on society through the efforts of those called on to treat them and the cost of providing health care for them. Does this mean that they are in fact causing harm to others and therefore that social direction of their behaviour is justified? For Mill, the answer seems to be clearly 'no':

> But with regard to the merely contingent, or, as it may be called, constructive injury which a person causes to society, by conduct which neither violates any specific duty to the public, nor occasions any perceptible hurt to any assignable individual except himself; the inconvenience is one which society can afford to bear, for the sake of the greater good of human freedom.
>
> (Mill, 1990: 213)

This position is contested, with proponents of stronger social intervention on issues such as tobacco and alcohol arguing that the overall cost of these behaviours for society justifies interference with individual liberties in this area. This is another area where different values come into conflict when considering specific issues of the politics and ethics of health promotion.

Activity 4.3

This activity encourages you to engage with the concept of liberalism in specific cases, and to identify some particular challenges.

1 What are the advantages and disadvantages of liberalism and only intervening where necessary to prevent harm to others? Consider how some specific health promotion issues would be addressed on this basis.
2 Mill argues that these freedoms only apply to adults 'in the maturity of their faculties' – how should others be treated?

Feedback

1 Advantages of this approach include *clarity*; this provides a clear test for when intervention is justified. It also respects the rights of the individual and avoids many of the
disadvantages of decisions by experts as described above.

The disadvantages include that this has quite significant *limits for health promotion*,
which frequently focuses on the good of the individual themselves, which is precisely
where Mill argues intervention is not justified. Moreover, even in cases where some
action causes harm to others but without intent and without harming a specific
individual (which might be the case for environmental damage, for example), Mill
seems to argue that intervention is not justified.

However, one important issue to note is that of *consent*. Following this approach
does not mean that health promotion aimed at the good of the individual cannot be
undertaken, only that it cannot be imposed without their agreement. As set out in
the first extract from *On Liberty*, Mill agrees that seeking the agreement of the
individual is reasonable; what Mill argues against is compelling someone against
their will for their own good. Thus the main limit on health promotion under this
approach comes from actions involving some element of obligation – in particular,
laws, regulations or other exercise of official authority.

2 This is also relevant for *children* and others who are not capable of making their own
decisions, for whatever reason; the key issue is that these people are not able to
decide for themselves what is in their own interest and thus there is a greater
responsibility on others to make those decisions for them. You should consider who
should make those decisions (such as parents or guardians for children) and why. Mill
also raises the issue of education and preparing children for life as adults and making
their own choices; your answer should address what kind of education would be
proper preparation from a health promotion perspective.

The four principles approach

Beauchamp and Childress (2009) defend what is termed the *four principles approach* to
health care ethics, also known by its opponents as *principalism*. The principles they
describe derive from 'considered judgements' in the common morality and medical
traditions. The four clusters of principles are:

1 *Respect for autonomy*: this requires respecting the decision-making capacities of
autonomous persons. Many philosophers agree that morality presupposes people
are able to act autonomously, but interpret this in different ways. Beauchamp and
Childress describe the autonomous individual as acting freely 'in accordance with a
self-chosen plan, analogous to the way an independent government manages its ter-
ritories and establishes its policies' (Beauchamp and Childress, 2009: 99). A 'person
of diminished autonomy, by contrast, is in some respect controlled by others or
incapable of deliberating or acting on the basis of his or her desires and plans' (ibid.).
Requiring informed consent for treatment is a well-established example of such
respect in individual health care, but this principle can also affect health promotion
questions. For example, one of the arguments in favour of the recent 'libertarian
paternalism' approach is that it can be used to promote health by altering default

options or other 'nudges' to promote health, but it does so while respecting the choices of individuals to do otherwise if they wish (Thaler and Sunstein, 2009).

2 *Non-maleficence*: avoiding the causation of harm. This is closely associated in medical ethics with the maxim *Primum non nocere*: 'Above all, do no harm'. In health care, a decision-making framework for situations that may involve life-sustaining procedures and assistance in dying, for example, is necessary. For health promotion, this might arise from unintended consequences of health promotion actions such as wider social effects of changes originally promoted to improve health, for example providing health information through channels that are accessed more by groups of higher socio-economic status, thus widening inequalities in health.

3 *Beneficence*: providing benefits and measuring benefits against risks and costs. Beauchamp and Childress (2009: 197) argue that 'principles of beneficence potentially demand much more than the principle of non-maleficence, because agents must take positive steps to help others, not merely refrain from harmful acts'. They describe two principles of beneficence: positive beneficence, meaning actively helping others, and utility, meaning balancing the different advantages, disadvantages, and costs to ensure the best overall outcome.

4 *Justice*: distributing benefits, risks, and costs fairly. Inequalities in health and access to health care are frequently raised as a moral problem in debates on social justice. This also links to much wider questions about rights to health, the role of government and public expenditure, socio-economic inequalities and their effect on health, individual freedom and our collective rights and obligations. Quite apart from differences in the resources of different countries, different societies have made quite different choices about what justice means for health, as shown clearly, for example, by the different approaches of the USA and European countries. Theoretical approaches to inequalities in health are discussed in more detail in Chapter 8.

In addition, Beauchamp and Childress describe three different types of rules that specify the four principles and serve as a guide to action. First, *substantive rules* include the rules of: telling the truth, confidentiality, privacy, fair allocation and rationing of health care, and so on. An example of a substantive rule that specifies the principle of respect for autonomy would be, 'Follow the wishes of the patient expressed in advance whenever they are clear and relevant.' Second, *authority rules* include the rules of *surrogate authority* (who should make decisions for incompetent persons), *professional authority* (who should assume responsibility for overriding or accepting patients' decisions in cases where these are potentially damaging), and *distributional authority* (who should make decisions about the distribution of resources). Third, *procedural rules* establish procedures to be followed when, for example, determining eligibility for medical resources or reporting grievances to higher authorities.

The market solution

Although the above four principles are a valuable guide for the specific issue of health promotion, they do not resolve the wider tensions between the different possible political approaches to resolving conflicting values. Is there a way of agreeing on a single common approach for philosophical principles underlying the relationship between individuals and wider society? In recent decades, the answer has increasingly come not from philosophers, but from another discipline – economics, and the use of markets to resolve different points of view.

Michael Sandel (2012) argues that there has been a trend in recent decades to replace discussions of ethics with the use of markets as an alternative philosophy, an approach sometimes described as 'neoliberalism'.

Why might the use of markets be problematic? Sandel argues that there are two fundamental problems, namely inequality and corruption. With inequalities in society come differences of purchasing power, but such differences can be more or less important depending on how many spheres of life are affected by those differences. The more societies structure our relations in all spheres of life as markets, though, the greater the impact of such inequalities. For health specifically, the impact of socio-economic inequalities is already clear, as for example described by the World Health Organization's Commission on Social Determinants of Health (CSDH, 2008).

With the second problem of corruption, Sandel is not referring so much to obvious issues of illicit payments, but rather the way in which treating something as a market commodity to be bought and sold changes the way in which we see it. It implies that what is being sold is something valued in monetary terms, but this may conflict with other values, which we think should apply instead.

Activity 4.4

In this activity, you will explore issues arising for the use of markets in health provision by looking at examples. One example Sandel describes is that of access to health care in China (Sandel, 2012: 24–5). Due to its limited availability in many areas, people travel to Beijing to seek health care. But rather than seeing people on the basis of their need, appointment tickets are sold; and then resold, with high prices to see leading specialists.

Another example that Sandel cites is that of 'Project Prevention', a project in the USA that offers cash incentives to people who are addicted to drugs if they will be sterilized or use long-term birth control (Sandel, 2012). This is argued to prevent harm to potential children who might be born to drug-addicted parents. It has also been criticized as being coercive, or as being corrupting. How would you analyse these different examples, and the arguments for and against them?

Feedback

Your analysis of the first example may raise obvious issues of inequality; it also says something about the nature of health care, as being not a response to medical need, but simply a commercial service. Your analysis of the second example is likely to show that this issue cannot only be analysed in economic terms of costs and benefits, but also requires a discussion of values. Issues of inequality and whether people who are addicted to drugs are in a position to make informed and free decisions about whether to accept such an offer are likely to be raised; this is again both an empirical question (about the impact of addiction on cognition, for example) and a question about values and power. You may also consider whether decisions about conception and children can be valued economically or whether a different kind of valuation is appropriate; and if so, whether these two types of value can co-exist, or whether applying an economic valuation in some way displaces other values.

Resolving political and ethical considerations in practice

As you will have seen, there is a wide range of possible approaches to considering political and ethical considerations. Each of these approaches is reflected to a certain extent in modern political discussion, without any of them being universally agreed. But there are also many other possible approaches. These include those based on religious beliefs. Religious belief can lead to a different perception of issues than a scientific approach, which can be particularly relevant for health care and other science-based disciplines.

This is not just a matter of philosophical discussion, however. It becomes an important question for health promotion, especially when carried out with or on behalf of public authorities or in pursuit of a public good. Health promotion by or on behalf of public authorities can involve some element of compulsion and even when it does not, it is often perceived as having a coercive element. It is thus important to have not just the agreement of individuals but also, where relevant, the agreement of society as a whole. Of course, there will be a general framework for political and ethical values expressed in the legal framework of the country concerned, which can be taken as describing the accepted rules for that environment. However, this is unlikely to address all the issues that can arise in health promotion. For example, the health impact of particular measures may be unclear or disputed. And even when the scientific evidence about the health consequences of a particular action are clear, individuals may still prefer to make choices that conflict with that advice. Health-related decisions may also conflict with other values (such as moral values) or other interests, requiring some means for making decisions.

To illustrate these issues, consider the following examples of political and ethical discussion over current issues in health promotion.

Measles, mumps, and rubella (MMR) vaccination

Controversy arose over this vaccine after a link with inflammatory bowel disease and autism was suggested in 1998. Despite broad scientific consensus that there is no evidence of a link between MMR and these conditions, public confidence in the safety of the vaccine was severely undermined and in the UK uptake declined by 8 per cent from the peak coverage of 92 per cent in 1995. The British Government decided not to provide vaccination for each of these conditions individually, citing increased danger both to the children concerned and to others through increased risk of transmission of these diseases, despite the concern of many parents over vaccination for their children with MMR.

Ban on smoking in public places

Several high-income countries have some form of ban on smoking in the workplace or public places, including Ireland, Norway, Malta, and some US states, citing the need to protect people (in particular workers) from the harmful effects of second-hand tobacco smoke. Proposals for such bans are often controversial and have been argued against on the grounds of the right of individuals to choose to smoke and the potential harm to commercial establishments from a fall in revenue due to smokers choosing to stay away. There have also been disputes between experts over how much harm second-hand tobacco smoke actually causes, although the balance of opinion appears to suggest that there is significant harm.

Health promotion as experimentation

As discussed in Chapter 3, the evidence base for different health promotion interventions may be unclear or disputed. Resources for health promotion are also often low. These challenges can be combined by carrying out experiments in health promotion – giving a certain intervention to some members of a potential target group but not others, and evaluating the results. Tim Harford gives the example of a Dutch charity funding money for treating children in Kenyan schools for intestinal worms. With limited funds, the charity opted to phase the intervention and use schools without the intervention for comparison (Harford, 2011). On the one hand, this can be argued to provide better evidence about how successful interventions really are. On the other hand, ethical concerns can be raised: Is it legitimate to conduct experiments in this way? Should limited resources not be targeted on those most in need, rather than used for comparisons?

Activity 4.5

This activity encourages you to bring together the different perspectives outlined during this chapter to see how they relate to practical issues.

1 What political and ethical issues do the above examples raise?
2 How could they best be resolved?

Feedback

1 These examples raise many of the issues already discussed in this chapter, such as the tension between expertise and individual choice, and between individual choices and the values of the community.

2 On the issue of MMR vaccination, your answer should identify issues around justifying action on scientific expertise and how to decide between expert judgements on the one hand and the wishes of individuals on the other when they conflict. This also raises issues about individual consent, as a government's decision not to offer the three separate vaccines can be considered to be, in effect, a form of official pressure, as well as the potential for harm to others through diseases transmitted due to lack of vaccination using MMR. You may also refer back to your answer under Activity 4.3 on how society should handle the health choices of children, as these vaccines are given at a young age and thus decisions are being made by parents or guardians.

On the issue of banning smoking in public places, this raises issues about the balance between individual consent and possible harm to others – also in terms of health, or sometimes in terms of other factors (such as the economic harm to commercial establishments). This is also a clear example of using political processes (legislation) to achieve a health promotion goal, including use of the coercive power of the state. You may have considered whether it is possible to compare different interests when they are of different types (such as by putting a monetary value on non-monetary interests to enable comparisons). This issue again raises questions about how to decide between different expert viewpoints, given the different views of experts over the harm from second-hand tobacco smoke.

The issue of health promotion as experimentation is likely to raise issues about ends and means, and whether the desirable end of producing good evidence justifies using an experimental approach in allocating resources or experimenting with different interventions; whether this implies treating the participants in the intervention as means rather than ends, and what this implies, perhaps referring back to Activity 4.4. You may make comparisons with clinical trials for health care interventions, which are a central part in licensing medicinal products, although these two have their own ethical dilemmas, and participation in clinical trials normally involves consent.

Summary

You have learnt about political and ethical aspects of health promotion, including identifying some of the political and ethical issues that health promotion may raise. You also learnt about five different approaches to considering political issues and the balances to be struck: a perfect society, described by Plato; utilitarianism; liberalism and individual freedom; the four principles approach; and how far there should be moral limits to markets. All of these approaches have advantages and disadvantages and the framework in which health promotion is carried out will involve elements of these and other approaches.

References

Beauchamp, T. and Childress, J. (2009) *Principles of Biomedical Ethics* (6th edn.). New York: Oxford University Press.

Commission on Social Determinants of Health (CSDH) (2008) *Closing the Gap in a Generation: Health Equity through Action on the Social Determinants of Health*. Final Report of the Commission on Social Determinants of Health. Geneva: WHO.

Harford, T. (2011) *Adapt: Why Success Always Starts with Failure*. London: Hachette Digital.

Mill, J. (1990) On Liberty, in M. Warnock (ed.) *Utilitarianism, On Liberty, Essay on Bentham: Together with Selected Writings of Jeremy Benthan and John Austin*. Glasgow: Collins/Fontana.

Plato (1989) The Republic, in E. Hamilton and H. Cairns (eds.) *The Collected Dialogues of Plato, including the Letters*. Princeton, NJ: Princeton University Press.

Sandel, M. (2012) *What Money Can't Buy: The Moral Limits of Markets*. London: Penguin.

Thaler, R.H. and Sunstein, C.R. (2009) *Nudge: Improving Decisions about Health, Wealth and Happiness* (illustrated, reprint edition). London: Penguin.

Further reading

Burns, J.H. and Hart, H.L.A. (eds.) (1977) *The Introduction to the Principles of Morals and Legislation*. London: Athline Press.

Cribb, A. and Duncan, P. (2002) *Health Promotion and Professional Ethics*. Oxford: Blackwell.

Elster, J. (1989) *Nuts and Bolts for the Social Sciences*. Cambridge: Cambridge University Press.

Norman, R. (1998) *The Moral Philosophers: An Introduction to Ethics* (2nd edn.). Oxford: Oxford University Press.

Sandel, M.J. (2012) *What Money Can't Buy: The Moral Limits of Markets*. London: Penguin.

Seedhouse, D. (1998) *Ethics: The Heart of Health Care* (2nd edn.). Chichester: Wiley.

SECTION 2

Using theory to inform health promotion practice

Using theory to guide change at the individual level

5

Don Nutbeam

Overview

This chapter provides an overview of the use of theory to guide health promotion directed at achieving change at the individual level, drawing upon some of the most influential theories and models that have guided health promotion practice in the recent past and which remain influential. When used thoughtfully, theories can greatly enhance the effectiveness and sustainability of health promotion programmes.

Learning objectives

After reading this chapter, you will be able to:

- identify ways in which the use of theory can help you understand the nature of the health problem being addressed, including the needs and motivations of the target population
- explain or make propositions concerning how to change health behaviours and social and environmental determinants of health
- recognize key measures used to monitor and evaluate a health promotion intervention

Key terms

Health behavior: Actions undertaken by an individual that have an effect (positive or negative) on health.

Self-efficacy: Belief in one's ability and capacity to achieve a goal.

Social determinants of health: The social, economic, and environmental factors which impact on health behaviours and determine the health status of individuals or populations.

Social norms: Pattern of behaviour in a particular group, community or culture, accepted as normal and to which an individual is expected to conform.

Theory: Systematically organized knowledge devised to analyse, predict or explain observable phenomena that could be used as the basis for action.

Introduction

Not all forms of public health intervention are equally successful in achieving their aims and objectives. Experience tells us that health promotion interventions are most likely to be successful when the determinants of a health problem or issue are well understood, where the needs and motivations of the target population are addressed, and the context in which the programme is being implemented has been taken into account.

Although many health promotion projects and programmes are developed and implemented without overt reference to theory, there is substantial evidence from published research demonstrating that the use of theory will significantly improve the chances of success in achieving pre-determined programme objectives (Glanz et al., 2008; Nutbeam et al., 2010).

Theory

Theory can be defined as systematically organized knowledge applicable in a relatively wide variety of circumstances devised to analyse, predict or otherwise explain the nature or behaviour of a specified set of phenomena that could be used as the basis for action (Van Ryn and Heany, 1992). A fully developed theory would explain:

- The major factors that influence the phenomena of interest, for example those factors that explain why some people are regularly physically active and others are not.
- The relationship between these factors, for example the relationship between knowledge, beliefs, social norms, and behaviours such as physical activity.
- The conditions under which these relationships do or do not occur. How, when, and why relationships exist, for example, the time, place and circumstances which, predictably, lead to a person being active or inactive.

Using theory in practice

Most health promotion theories come from the behavioural and social sciences. They borrow from disciplines such as psychology and sociology and from activities such as management, consumer behaviour, and marketing. Such diversity reflects the fact that health promotion practice is not only concerned with the behaviour of individuals but also with the ways in which society is organized and the policies and organizational structures that underpin social organization.

Many of the theories commonly used in health promotion are not highly developed in the way suggested in the definition above, nor have they been rigorously tested when compared, for example, with theory in the physical sciences. For these reasons, many of the theories referred to below are more accurately termed 'models'.

The potential of theory to guide the development of health promotion interventions is substantial. There are several different planning models that are used by health promotion practitioners. Internationally, among the best known of these planning models is the PRECEDE/PROCEED model developed by Green and Kreuter (2005), and the RE-AIM framework developed by Glasgow and colleagues (1999). Several variations of this approach have also been produced, often in an attempt to incorporate better the social and environmental determinants of health than the established models.

In each case, these models and guidelines follow a structured sequence, including planning, implementation, and evaluation. Reference to different theories can guide and inform practitioners at each of these stages. Figure 5.1 provides a summary of the key phases in the process, and examples of the different elements, actions, and indicators that can be used to shape programme planning, implementation, and evaluation.

The use of theory in each of these stages is considered in turn.

Problem definition

Identification of the parameters of the health problem to be addressed may involve drawing on a wide range of epidemiological and demographic information, as well as information from available sources on health-related behaviours, social, economic and environmental conditions, and knowledge of community needs and priorities. Here, different theories can help you identify *what* should be the focus for an intervention.

Specifically, theory can inform your choice for the focus for the intervention. This may be the individual characteristics, beliefs, and values that are associated with different health behaviours and that may be amenable to change. Alternatively, the focus might be on social or environmental conditions that may need to be changed.

Solution generation

The second step involves the analysis of potential solutions, leading to the development of a programme plan that specifies the objectives and strategies to be employed, as well as the sequence of activity. Theory is at its most useful here in providing guidance on *how* and *when* change might be achieved in the target population, organization or policy. It may also generate ideas that might not otherwise have occurred to you.

Different theories can help you understand the methods you could use as the focus of your interventions; specifically by improving understanding of the processes by which changes occur in the target variables (i.e. people, organizations, and policies), and by clarifying the means of achieving change in these target variables. For example, *theory* may help explain the influence of different social influences, or environmental conditions and their impact on individual behavioural choices. These insights will help in the design of a programme, for example by indicating how changes to the environment can have an impact on health behaviour.

Thus, those theories that explain and predict individual and group health behaviour and organizational practice, as well as those that identify methods for changing these determinants of health behaviour and organizational practice, are worthy of close consideration in this phase of planning. Some theories also inform decisions on the timing and sequencing of your interventions in order to achieve maximum effects.

Capacity building

Once a programme plan has been developed, the first phase in implementation is usually directed towards generating public and political interest in the programme,

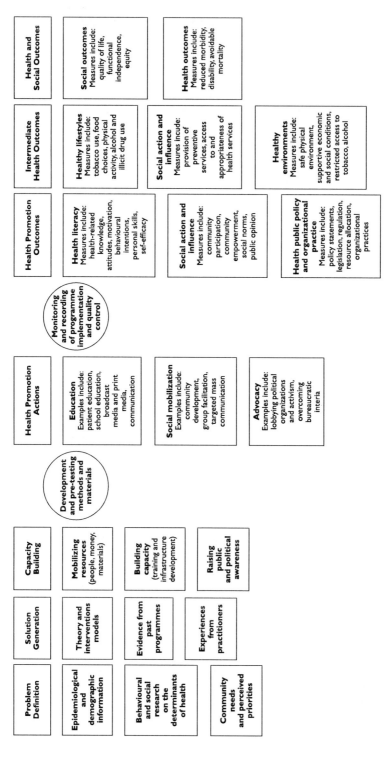

Figure 5.1 A planning model for health promotion. In now out of print book Nutbeam, D. (2001) Effective health promotion programmes, in Pencheon D, Guest C, Meltzer, D, Muir, Gray, J.A. (eds.) Oxford Handbook of Public Health Practice. Reproduced by permission of Oxford University Press

mobilizing resources for programme implementation, and building capacity in organizations through which the programme may operate (e.g. schools, worksites, local government). Models and theories that indicate how to influence organizational policy and procedures are particularly useful here, as too is *theory* that guides the development and use of different media, including, for example, the social media.

Health promotion actions

The implementation of a programme may involve multiple strategies, such as education and social mobilization. Here, the key elements of theory can provide a benchmark against which *actual* selection of methods and sequencing of an intervention can be considered in relation to the *theoretically* ideal implementation of programmes.

In practice, it is not always possible to do what may be theoretically ideal. The use of theory helps you to understand observed success or failure in different programmes by highlighting the possible impact of differences between what was planned and what actually happened in the implementation of the programme. It can also assist in identifying and describing the key elements of a programme that can form the basis for disseminating successful programmes.

Evaluating outcomes

Health promotion interventions can be expected to have an impact initially on processes or activities such as personal and community participation, organizational practices, and even government policies. Theory can provide guidance on the appropriate measures that can be used to assess such activities. For example, where theory suggests that the target of interventions is to achieve a specific change in knowledge about something (for example, healthy weight), or changes in social attitudes towards something (such as smoking), measurement of these changes becomes the first point of evaluation. Such impact measures are often referred to as *health promotion outcomes* (see Figure 5.1).

Intermediate outcome assessment is the next level of evaluation. Theory can also be used to predict the *intermediate health outcomes* that are sought from an intervention. Usually these are modifications of people's behaviour or changes in social, economic, and environmental conditions that determine health or influence behaviour. For example, theories can predict the ways in which changes in knowledge, motivations, and intentions will lead to changes in health behaviours.

Health and social outcomes refer to the final outcomes of an intervention in terms of changes in physical or mental health status, in quality of life, or in improved equity in health within populations. Definition of final outcomes will be based on theoretically predicted relationships between changes in intermediate health outcomes (behaviours and social conditions) and final health outcomes.

Table 5.1 summarizes the areas of change and some of the theories or models underpinning them to support the planning, execution, and evaluation of health promotion programmes. This chapter introduces you to some important theories used to guide individual behaviour change. Others are described elsewhere in this book.

Table 5.1 Areas of change and the theories or models underpinning them. From Nutbeam, D., Harris, E., Wise, M. (2010) Theory in a Nutshell: A Practical Guide to Health Promotion Theories. Reproduced by permission of McGraw-Hill.

Areas of change	Theories or models
Theories that explain health behaviour and health behaviour change by focusing on the individual	• Health belief model • Theory of reasoned action • Transtheoretical (stages of change) model • Social learning theory

Theories that explain change in communities and community action for health	• Community mobilization
	  – Social planning
	  – Social action
	  – Community development
	• Diffusion of innovation

Theories that guide the use of communication strategies for change to promote health	• Communication for behaviour change • Social marketing
Models that explain changes in organizations and the creation of health-supportive organizational practices	• Theories of organizational change • Models of intersectoral action
Models that explain the development and implementation of healthy public policy	• Framework for healthy public policy – health in all policies • Health impact assessment

Source: Nutbeam et al. (2010)

Selecting an appropriate theory

Theories are not static pronouncements that can be applied to all issues in all circumstances. In health promotion, some of the theories used have been extensively refined and developed in the light of experience, while others are 'work in progress', less well-developed ideas subject to continuous refinement. The range of theories used in health promotion has expanded over the past two decades from a focus on the modification of individual behaviour, to recognition of the need to influence and change a broad range of social, organizational, and environmental factors that influence health alongside individual behavioural choices.

Choosing the right approach is moderated by the nature of the problem, its determinants, and the opportunities for action. Programmes that operate at multiple levels, such as those envisaged by the Ottawa Charter for Health Promotion (WHO, 1986) are more likely to address the full range of determinants of health problems in populations, and thereby have the greatest effect.

Activity 5.1

In this activity, you will consider the wide range of different actions and interventions that can be used in health promotion. Consider a programme to improve the uptake of a childhood immunization in your country. Suggest some interventions that could be implemented with individual parents, a whole local community, the organization of services, and the whole population at the national level.

Feedback

Possible interventions could include:

- *For individual parents*: education to inform and motivate individual parents to immunize their children.
- *For the local community*: facilitation of community debate to change social perceptions concerning the safety and convenience of immunization, and social norms concerning the need for immunization.
- *For the organization of services*: changes to organizational practice to improve reminder and notification systems for parents and provide more conveniently located clinics.
- *At the national level*: policy change providing financial (or other material) incentives for parents and doctors to immunize children.

It follows that no single theory dominates health promotion practice and nor could it, given the range of health problems and their determinants, the diversity of populations and settings, and differences in available resources, skills, and opportunity for action among practitioners.

Depending on the level of an intervention (individual, group, organization or nation) and the type of change (simple, one-off behaviour, complex behaviour, organizational or policy change), different theories will have greater relevance and provide a better fit with the problem. None of the theories or models presented in this book can simply be adopted as the answer to all problems. Most often, you benefit by drawing upon more than one of the theories to match the multiple levels of the programme being contemplated.

To be useful and relevant, the different models and theories have to be readily understood and capable of application in a wide variety of real-life conditions. Although we are constantly reminded that 'there is nothing so practical as a good theory', we may remain somewhat suspicious of the capacity of intervention theories to provide the guidance necessary to develop an effective intervention in a complex environment.

Theories and models are simplified representations of reality – they can never include or explain all of the complexities of individual, social or organizational behaviour. However, while the use of theory alone does not guarantee effective programmes, the use of theory in the planning, implementation, and evaluation of programmes will enhance the chances of success. One of the greatest challenges for you is to identify how best to achieve a fit between the issues of interest and established theories or models, which could improve the effectiveness of a programme or intervention.

Theoretical models for individual health behaviour change

One of the major roots of health promotion can be found in the application of health psychology to health behaviour change. Evidence for this can be seen in the phenomenal growth in the discipline of health psychology and the evolution of the concept of behavioural medicine in the past 20 years. This discipline has had a significant influence. For several decades researchers have sought to explain, predict, and change health behaviour through the development and application of theories and models evolving from psychology and, in particular, social psychology. Let us now explore three theories that have been proposed to explain individual health behaviour.

The health belief model

This is one of the longest established theoretical models designed to explain health behaviour by understanding people's beliefs about health. It was originally articulated to explain why individuals participate in health screening and immunization programmes, and has been developed for application to other types of health behaviour.

At its core, the model suggests that the likelihood of an individual taking action for a given health problem is based on the interaction between four types of belief (Figure 5.2). The model predicts that individuals will take action to protect or promote health if:

- they perceive themselves to be susceptible to a condition or problem
- they believe it will have potentially serious consequences
- they believe a course of action is available that will reduce their susceptibility, or minimize the consequences
- they believe that the benefits of taking action will outweigh the costs or barriers.

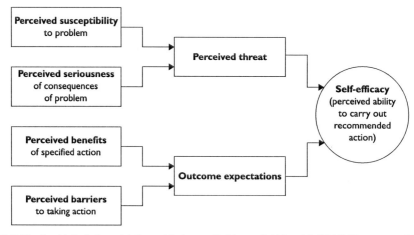

Figure 5.2 The health belief model. From Nutbeam, D., Harris, E., Wise, M. (2010) Theory in a Nutshell: A Practical Guide to Health Promotion Theories. Reproduced by permission of McGraw-Hill.

Activity 5.2

In this activity, you will consider the practical application of the health belief model in health promotion. Imagine you are developing a public education programme for HIV prevention in your country. List the beliefs necessary for people to adopt behaviour change to minimize their risk of infection according to the health belief model. If it is helpful, target the project to a particular population group (such as adolescents, or sex workers).

Feedback

Individuals would need to:

- believe that they are at risk of HIV infection
- believe that the consequences of infection are serious
- receive supportive cues for action which may trigger a response (such as targeted media publicity)
- believe that risk minimization practices (such as safe sex or abstinence) will greatly reduce the risk of infection
- believe that the benefits of action to reduce risk will outweigh potential costs and barriers, such as reduced enjoyment and negative reactions of their partner
- believe in their ability to take effective action, such as following and maintaining safe sex behaviours.

Studies have shown how something as simple as the use of a postcard to remind parents of immunizations that are due for their children are effective in raising immunization rates. Hawe and colleagues (1998) compared the difference in impact on immunization rates between using the health belief model to guide the content of a simple postcard message to encourage parents to bring their children for immunization and that of a standard card that provided only the time and place of the immunization clinic. This simple modification, guided by the health belief model, produced a significant improvement in the uptake of immunization in the community in which it was tested.

Generally, the health belief model has been found to be most useful when applied to behaviours for which it was originally developed, particularly prevention strategies such as screening and immunization. It has been less useful in guiding interventions to address more long-term, complex, and socially determined behaviours, such as alcohol and tobacco consumption. The model's advantage is the relatively simple way in which it illustrates the importance of individual beliefs about health and the relative costs and benefits of actions to protect or improve health. Three decades of research have indicated that promoting change in beliefs can lead to changes in health behaviour that contribute to improved health status. Changes in knowledge and beliefs will almost always form part of a health promotion programme, and the health belief model provides a reference point in the development of messages to improve knowledge and change beliefs using print, electronic, and other mass media.

The stages of change (transtheoretical) model

Prochaska and DiClemente (1984) developed this model to describe and explain the different stages in behaviour change. The model is based on the premise that behaviour change is a process, not an event, and that individuals have different levels of motivation or readiness to change. Five stages of change, which are shown in Figure 5.3, have been identified:

- *Precontemplation*: this describes individuals who are not even considering changing behaviour or are consciously intending not to change.
- *Contemplation*: the stage at which a person considers making a change to a specific behavior.

- *Determination* (or preparation): the stage at which a person makes a serious commitment to change.
- *Action*: the stage at which behaviour change is initiated.
- *Maintenance*: sustaining the change, and achievement of predictable health gains. *Relapse* may also be the fifth stage.

From a programme planning perspective, the model is particularly useful in indicating how different *processes of change* can influence how activities are staged. Several processes have been consistently useful in supporting movement between stages. These processes are more or less applicable at different stages of change. For example, awareness-raising may be most useful among pre-contemplators who may not be aware of the threat to health that their behaviour poses, whereas communication of the benefits of change and illustration of the success of others in changing may be important for those contemplating change. Once change has been initiated at the

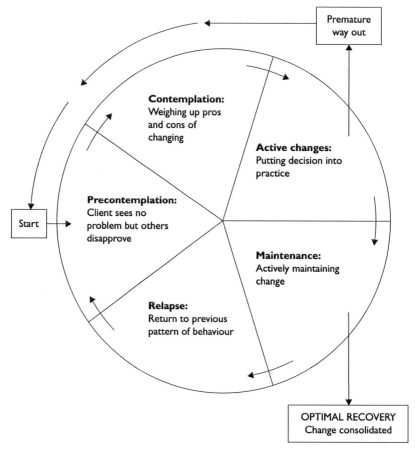

Figure 5.3 The stages of change (transtheoretical) model. From Prochaska, J.O., DiClemente, C.C. (1984) The Transtheoretical Approach: Crossing Traditional Boundaries of Therapy. Reproduced by permission of Dow Jones Irwin.

action stage, social support and stimulus control (for example, by avoiding certain situations or having environmental supports in place) are more important.

By matching stages of behavioural change with specific processes, the model specifies how interventions could be organized for different populations, with different needs and in different circumstances. The stages of change model stresses the need to research the characteristics of the target population, the importance of not assuming that all people are at the same stage, and the need to organize interventions sequentially to address the different stages that will be encountered.

The model has been applied in a wide variety of settings, and to address a range of behaviours and conditions. For example, it has been used in a workplace programme to promote regular physical activity and stress management – interventions that traditionally have met with limited success. Prochaska and colleagues (2008) tested an intervention that used the stages of change model to tailor interventions to workers' current level of activity and motivation to change. The intervention consisted of a transtheoretical tailored communication (TTM), motivational interviewing (MI), and a brief health risk intervention (HRI) in a worksite sample according to the different stage of change. The intervention produced promising short-term results by supporting many participants to move on through the different stages of change towards more regular activity and effective risk management.

Activity 5.3

In this activity, you will consider the practical application of the transtheoretical model. Identify three different forms of intervention that would assist individuals in weight control, moving from their current stage of change to the next stage.

Feedback

There are many forms of intervention you may have suggested. For example, in the contemplation stage, information and advice on the health problems associated with being overweight, and the feasibility of losing weight might help a patient move from the *pre-contemplation* to the *contemplation* stage. Developing an individual, tailored plan for weight loss and providing a mechanism for feedback may help tip the 'decisional balance' from the *determination* to the *action* stage. Improving access to gym facilities, and providing healthy food options in a worksite canteen may help with the longer term *maintenance* of optimal weight.

The stages of change model has become an important reference point in health promotion interventions because of its obvious advantage in focusing on the change process. The model is important in emphasizing the range of needs for an intervention in any given population, the changing needs of different populations, and the need for the sequencing of interventions to match different stages of change. It illustrates the importance of tailoring programmes to the real needs and circumstances of individuals, rather than assuming an intervention will be equally applicable to all. As Activity 5.3 illustrates, it can also prompt consideration of a wide range of interventions.

However, a recent review of findings from health behaviour interventions using the transtheoretical model (Bridle et al., 2005) found mixed evidence of effectiveness from studies of 'highly variable quality'. The model has been criticized for failing to account for the full complexity of behavioural change processes. Although it has been proposed as a model that serves as an umbrella for other theories that guide health promotion practice, its strong roots in behavioural psychology and primary application in clinical settings with individuals makes this assessment somewhat optimistic. It may be best considered as a useful approach to defining needs and structuring interventions to improve the health of individuals.

Social cognitive theory

This is one of the most widely applied theories in health promotion because it addresses both the underlying determinants of health behaviour and the methods of promoting change. The theory was built on an understanding of the interaction that occurs between an individual and their environment (Bandura, 1995). Early psycho-social research tended to focus on the way in which an environment shapes behaviour, by making it more or less rewarding to behave in particular ways. For example, if at work there is no regulation on where people are able to smoke cigarettes, it is easy to be a smoker. If regulations are in place, it is more difficult and, as a consequence, most smokers smoke less and find such an environment more supportive for quitting.

Social cognitive theory indicates that the relationship between people and their environment is more subtle and complex. For example, in circumstances where a significant number of people are non-smokers and are assertive about their desire to restrict smoking in a given environment, even without formal regulation, it becomes far less rewarding for the individual who smokes. They are then likely to modify their behaviour. In this case, the non-smokers have influenced the smoker's perception of the environment through social influence.

This is referred to as 'reciprocal determinism'. It describes the way in which an individual, their environment, and behaviour continuously interact and influence each other. An understanding of this interaction and the way in which modification of social norms can impact on behaviour offers an important insight into how behaviour can be modified through health promotion interventions. For example, seeking to modify social norms regarding smoking is considered to be one of the most powerful ways of promoting cessation among adults.

In addition to this basic understanding of the relationship between the individual and the environment, a range of personal cognitive factors form a third part of this relationship, affecting and being affected by specific behaviours and environments. Of these cognitions, three are particularly important. The first of these is the capacity to learn by observing both the behaviour of others and the rewards received for different patterns of behaviour. This is termed 'observational learning'. For example, some young women may observe behaviour (such as smoking) by people whom they regard as sophisticated and attractive so use as *role models*. If they observe and value the rewards that they associate with smoking, such as personal attractiveness or a desirable self-image, they are more likely to smoke themselves – their expectancies in relation to smoking are positive. Such an understanding further reinforces the importance of taking account of peer influences and social norms on health behaviour, and of the potential use of role models in influencing social norms.

The second of these cognitions is the capacity to anticipate and place value on the outcome of different behaviour patterns, referred to as 'expectations'. For example, if you believe that smoking will help you lose weight and you place great value on losing weight, then you are more likely to take up or to continue smoking. This understanding emphasizes the importance of understanding personal beliefs and motivations underlying different behaviour, and the need to emphasize short-term and tangible benefits. For example, young people have been shown to respond far more to the short-term adverse effects of smoking, such as bad breath and smelly clothes, than to any long-term threat posed to health by lung cancer or heart disease.

The final cognition the theory emphasizes is the importance of belief in your own ability to successfully perform a behaviour, referred to as 'self-efficacy'. Self-efficacy is proposed as the most important prerequisite for behaviour change and will affect how much effort is put into a task and the outcome of that task. The promotion of self-efficacy is thus an important task in the achievement of behaviour change. It has been proposed that both observational learning and participatory learning (for example, by supervised practice and repetition) will lead to the development of the knowledge and skills necessary for behaviour change, known as 'behavioural capability'. These are seen as powerful tools in building self-confidence and self-efficacy.

Taken as a whole, social cognitive theory provides a comprehensive and integrated theoretical basis for health promotion programmes. It recognizes the fundamental importance of individual beliefs, values, and self-confidence in determining health behaviour, as does the health belief model. It also explicitly identifies the importance of social norms and cues (social modelling) and environmental influences on health behaviour, and the continuous interaction between these variables.

Social cognitive theory also provides practical direction on how to modify these influences. In addition, this model suggests a different role for the practitioner who becomes a 'change agent', facilitating change through modification of the social environment and development of self-efficacy in ways that enable individuals to act to improve their health. Furthermore, it assists in understanding the multiple levels at which a health promotion programme may need to work. The application of this model can be seen in health promotion interventions that combine educational programmes with modification of the social and physical environments.

Activity 5.4

In this activity, you will look at the practical application of social cognitive theory. Using the three key cognitions from social cognitive theory, identify the key components of a programme to reduce the uptake of smoking among teenagers in your country.

Feedback

There are many types of action suggested by social cognitive theory. Examples include:

- using the mass media (especially social media) to change social norms regarding the acceptability of smoking
- using role models (for example, from sports, fashion or music) to advocate non-smoking
- changing expectations in relation to smoking by emphasizing short-term consequences of smoking such as bad breath and smelly clothes
- working with young people in formal settings (such as the classroom) to help them to develop self-efficacy in resisting peer pressures to smoke.

Summary

You have learnt about the importance of theory in health promotion and how to apply theory in the design and delivery of health promotion activities. Theories that focus on the individual provide important guidance on major elements of health promotion programmes. Taken together, the theories and models described in this chapter emphasize the importance of knowledge and beliefs about health, the importance of self-efficacy (the belief in one's competency to take action), the importance of perceived social norms and social influences related to the value an individual places on social approval or acceptance by different social groups, and the importance of recognizing that individuals in a population may be at different stages of change at any one time. However, as this chapter has outlined, there are limitations to psychosocial theories which do not adequately take account of socio-economic and environmental conditions. Consequently, changing these conditions or people's perception of these conditions is important if health promotion activities are to be effective.

References

Bandura, A. (1995) *Self-efficacy in Changing Societies*. New York: Cambridge University Press.

Bridle, C., Riemsma, R.P., Pattenden, J., Sowden, A.J., Mather, L., Watt, I.S. et al. (2005) Systematic review of the effectiveness of health behavior interventions based on the transtheoretical model, *Psychology and Health*, 20(3): 283–301.

Glanz, K., Rimer, B.K. and Viswanath, K. (2008) *Health Behaviour and Health Education: Theory, Research and Practice*. San Francisco, CA: Jossey-Bass.

Glasgow, R.E., Vogt, T.M. and Boles, S.M. (1999) Evaluating the public health impact of health promotion interventions: the RE-AIM framework, *American Journal of Public Health*, 89(9): 1322–7.

Green, L.W. and Kreuter, M.W. (2005) *Health Promotion Planning: An Educational and Ecological Approach*. Mountain View, CA: Mayfield.

Hawe, P., McKenzie, N. and Scurry, R. (1998) Randomised controlled trial of the use of a modified postal reminder card on the uptake of measles vaccination, *Archives of Disease in Childhood*, 79: 136–40.

Nutbeam, D. (2001) Effective health promotion programmes, in D. Pencheon, C. Guest, D. Meltzer and J.A. Muir Gray (eds.) *Oxford Handbook of Public Health Practice*. Oxford: Oxford University Press.

Nutbeam, D., Harris, E. and Wise, M. (2010) *Theory in a Nutshell: A Practical Guide to Health Promotion Theories*. Sydney, NSW: McGraw-Hill.

Prochaska, J.O. and DiClemente, C.C. (1984) *The Transtheoretical Approach: Crossing Traditional Boundaries of Therapy*. Homewood, IL: Dow Jones Irwin.

Prochaska, J.O., Butterworth, S., Redding, C.A., Burden, V., Perrin, N., Leo, M. et al. (2008) Initial efficacy of MI, TTM tailoring and HRI's with multiple behaviors for employee health promotion, *Preventive Medicine*, 46(3): 226–31.

Van Ryn, M. and Heany, C.A. (1992) What's the use of theory?, *Health Education Quarterly*, 19(3): 315–30.

World Health Organization (WHO) (1986) *Ottawa Charter for Health Promotion*. Geneva: WHO.

Using theory to guide change at the community level

6

Morten Skovdal

Overview

Those concerned with health promotion tend to target their efforts at various levels, from global, national and regional levels down to community and individual levels. Each level is important and health promotion practitioners should look to harmonize these multi-level efforts. The community is the crossroads between these levels. Communities translate health promotion messages and promote social cohesion – shaping our lived experiences and the way we conduct ourselves, including our health behaviours. Understanding how to engage with local communities to provide more health-enabling social environments is therefore key to health promotion theory. For these reasons, this chapter focuses on the health-promoting role of the community as a pathway for change.

Learning objectives

After reading this chapter, you will be able to:

- explain the relevance and role of community level structures in promoting health
- draw on conceptual perspectives to understand how health promoters can help guide change at a community level for improved health
- identify ways to better integrate health programmes into a social context and facilitate community responses for health

Key terms

Community capacity building: Enabling people in communities to participate in actions based on community interests.

Community health competence: The degree to which a community is health-enabling and responsive.

Community response: The combination of actions and steps taken by community members for the public good, including the provision of goods and services.

Conscientization: The development of a critical consciousness, a better understanding of the inequalities that exist in the world, particularly in relation to self.

Participatory learning and action: An approach for learning about and engaging with communities using participatory and visual methods to facilitate a process of collective learning and action.

Salutogenesis: An approach focusing on factors that support human health and well-being, rather than on factors that cause disease.

Social capital: The social benefits that derive from social networks and collaboration between people, and their shared values and norms of behaviour.

Introduction

As Section 1 of this book explored, the 1986 Ottawa Charter built on the Declaration of Alma Ata and the Health for All philosophy by redefining the field of health promotion. It did so by encouraging a shift away from a focus on the modification of individuals and their health-damaging behaviours to recognizing the importance of the social environment in shaping and determining health actions. This is because an individual's decision to engage in health-damaging behaviours, such as smoking or refusing to use a condom, are not necessarily determined by rational thinking of the risk factors, even if the knowledge is there. Instead, they are influenced by the extent to which the social environment supports, or even encourages, such behaviours (Campbell, 2001). Individuals do not live in a vacuum but in social and community contexts that have the potential to enable, or inhibit, health-enhancing behaviours. This is a paradigm shift that has changed the role of health promoters working at a community level. Health promotion at a community level is no longer about 'experts' providing target audiences with health-related information, but is about engaging with local actors to challenge health-damaging practices and norms as well as to facilitate locally defined solutions to health problems. However, a real shift has been slow because didactic and information-based health promotion methods are relatively straightforward and easy to get off the ground compared with engagement and facilitation approaches. Furthermore, there is limited understanding of theories guiding change at a community level.

What do we mean by community level?

Health promotion practitioners working at a community level are faced with the challenge of having to define what is meant by community in the context of their work. Often community refers to a geographically bounded area, a neighbourhood or a village. While this is a relatively simple understanding of community, it becomes more complicated when the definition is expanded to include members who share a common social identification. This understanding of community recognizes that individuals belong to a number of communities, both within a geographical area and beyond, each of which can play a health-enabling or -inhibiting role. A community of identity may include a group of people who share a set of beliefs and history (for example, a religious community), a sexual identity (for example, gay men), experiences of marginalization and discrimination (for example, people living with a stigmatized disease), hobbies and interests (for example, a sports club, or online gamers forming a virtual community), or a a common purpose which collectively they work towards (for example, women's groups). These and other social groupings form communities of people with common experiences, interests or beliefs. People are likely to actively participate in and draw on the benefits of a number of different social groupings at any one time. How these communities are experienced, as well as their significance for health, differ markedly and may come down to the nature of the social interaction that binds people together.

Activity 6.1

This activity encourages you to reflect on the diversity of community. What communities are you a part of? Make a list of all the communities you think you belong to. Think about what qualifies you to be a member of these communities and how each of those communities plays a role in facilitating your health and well-being.

Feedback

Your examples will show how diverse communities are, how they overlap, and how they influence behaviour.

Although the Internet has enabled social interaction to transcend beyond the locality of people, most social interaction still takes place in local social environments, and as such, the spatial dimension of community remains significant. Community level in this chapter therefore refers to the local social environment where norms, local institutions, and social interaction (often in 'communities of identity') mediate responses to health.

Health-enabling social environments

As discussed in Section 1 of this book, the field of health promotion has moved beyond a focus on individual behaviour and recognizes the importance of a wide range of social and environmental interventions. The role of community level health promoters is therefore to facilitate the process of health-enabling social environments, where people are in a position to take control over – and improve – their own health and that of others. Consequently, community participation and empowerment are key to community health promotion. Before discussing theories that can guide change at a community level, it is useful to describe some of the social structures, actors, and contexts that are part of a health-enabling social environment and thus play a key facilitating or inhibiting role in health promotion at a community level.

A model often used in the field of health promotion to discuss pathways to more health-enabling social environments, and the interplay between social structures, is the social ecological model (Bronfenbrenner, 1979; Stokols, 1996). The model, as illustrated in Figure 6.1, usefully situates the community within a broader and vertical context, locating the community at the intersection between individuals and their immediate family and wider socio-political and cultural factors, thus playing a key role in mediating

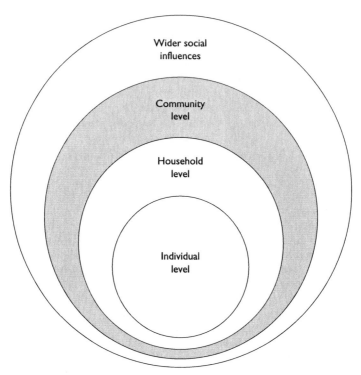

Figure 6.1 The social ecological model
Source: Adapted from Bronfenbrenner (1979)

initiatives for improved health. What the model highlights is that changes at a community level are inter-dependent on wider social influences. Empowerment and health-
enabling behaviours do not happen in a vacuum. More specifically, contexts enable, and
in some cases inhibit, the effectiveness of community level responses to health promotion. This means it is essential to consider wider social influences in community level
health promotion. These contexts include the availability of material (for example, condoms or sustained funding from global actors), symbolic factors (for example, social
policies being aligned with local realities or gender constructions), relational issues (for
example, patient–nurse relationships, level of community involvement), and institutional
factors (for example, the quality and availability of health services) (Campbell and
Cornish, 2010; Skovdal et al., 2011a, 2011b).

Nonetheless, it is at a community level that health promotion initiatives take shape
and get appropriated to local realities. It is at a community level where identities are
created as well as where social knowledge, shared meanings, and common values get
enacted – with the capacity to influence health-related behaviours both positively and
negatively. It is at a community level where health-related behaviours are learned and
practised, affirming the intrinsically social connection to health.

Playing an active role in shaping these norms, values, and health-related behaviours
are smaller level and inter-dependent social structures horizontally nested within the
community level. These social structures make up tangible actors, representing a
mix of external change agents, such as local non-governmental organizations, local

government departments, schools and churches and indigenous community groups, networks and other 'communities of identity'. Learning how to engage with and empower these social structures is pivotal to community level health promotion.

The field of health promotion is dominated by formal responses that enable people to take control over, and to improve, their health. Here, health promotion initiatives, spearheaded by more technical and resourceful organizations, involve community members in their programme design and implementation. While this continues to be important and integral to health promotion initiatives, there is also a need to acknowledge that most responses to health continue to be led by local community groups and networks, often with no support from external change agents. This is particularly the case in countries where health care is not a public good. This can be exemplified by the community response to HIV in Africa. Here indigenous community resources (such as community norms, networks, connectedness, assets, critical consciousness, and opportunities for dialogue) have been observed to, although not always, provide significant 'behind the scenes' support for those living with or affected by HIV (Campbell et al., in press; Gregson et al., in press). Indigenous community responses can therefore have a positive impact on behaviour change and much can be learned from them to strengthen and align more formal community level health promotion initiatives with local resources. A recognition of indigenous community responses also paves the way for the opportunity for health promotion not only to be about enabling individuals to take control over their health, but also to be about enabling community members to play a role in improving the health of others.

Against this background, to facilitate effective health-enabling social environments, health promoters working at a community level must recognize and bridge local *and* global structures responding to health, establishing dialogue between local community members and global actors penetrating local communities. Health promoters working at a community level must serve as mediators and make every effort to understand the context in which they work and identify key actors and contextual factors facilitating or inhibiting health and well-being. Health promoters can use this information to work with local community structures to devise a strategy that establishes productive alliances that can work towards the building of health-enabling social environments. Echoing the above, Figure 6.2 details a pyramid that outlines some questions that health promoters working at a community level can ask to gain a better understanding of the social structures, factors, and contexts that impact change at a community level. This information can be used to identify pathways towards a more health-enabling social environment and can inform a theory of change.

Why do we need a theory of change?

Theories of change help us unpack pathways to change. They are often advanced by social scientists and applied by practitioners. They make explicit the role of health promoters and uncover the thinking and beliefs that guide our assumptions of how interventions can make an impact. A theory of change articulates what activities have to occur for an expected change to happen. Put simply, by doing x (an action), y (a change) will be achieved. Needless to say, no social change initiative is that straightforward, and most mature theories of change are made up of systematically organized knowledge that provides you with a comprehensive road map to consider the populations you are serving, and help you establish the broader context and other major factors influencing

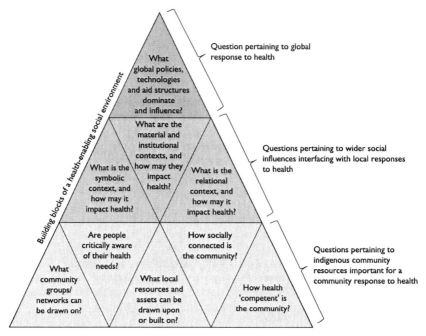

Figure 6.2 Questions to consider when developing a community level health promotion strategy

change. Mapping out the preconditions influencing pathways to change can help circumvent failure and optimize the impact of a health promotion strategy.

Moreover, a theory of change can crystallize the intended results of a social change initiative and that way help practitioners plan and develop health promotion strategies that can be evaluated. A theory of change can thus become a useful tool in demonstrating success and lessons learned.

Activity 6.2

In this activity, you will analyse how theories of change apply in practice. In rural Zimbabwe, some men fail to make use of HIV testing and treatment services. Local understandings of what it means to be a 'real man' appear to conflict with the expectations of users of HIV services. For example, some men in parts of rural Zimbabwe do not want to accept that they are vulnerable and at risk of contracting HIV, and those living with HIV are given lessons (often by female nurses) on how to live healthily, requesting them to stop engaging in certain activities (such as drinking alcohol and extramarital sex) that some men participate in to project and exert their masculinity (Skovdal et al., 2011a). Against your interest to improve HIV service use by men in this context, develop your own theory of change by asking the following two questions:

1 What change would you like to see happen so that men in this context are more likely to make use of HIV services?
2 What must happen in this context for your change to be realized?

Feedback

Your change should be plausible and focus on changes in and between people and groups that a social change initiative can realistically tackle, for example, make men feel more at ease with HIV and HIV services. Your vision should not point to an idealized and unachievable state such as transforming local understandings of masculinity. Your vision should be dynamic, and reflect the complexity of the social structures in which the initiative would be located.

Your actions, or pre-conditions for change, can either consist of tangible changes (for example, male-friendly HIV services such as men-only clinics, male nurses, peer support groups for men) or process outcomes (for example, attitude changes, more lenient and flexible understandings of masculinity, supportive relationships and confidence as a result of community conversations, peer group meetings or community role models discussing the impact of masculinity on HIV service use).

In the field of health promotion there is growing recognition of the need to learn from pathways to achievement and health as a way to guide theories of change. For example, a theory of change to address men's inclination to use HIV services could be strengthened by knowing how some men manage to construct HIV-service-friendly masculinities and successfully adhere to anti-retroviral therapy without feeling social pressure to conform to hegemonic and local understandings of manhood.

Conceptual perspectives and theories guiding change at a community level

There are a host of theories and conceptual frameworks that seek to explain, predict, and change pathways towards more health-enabling social environments. In this section, you will learn about four key conceptual perspectives that will advance your understanding of possibilities for change at a community level.

Critical consciousness and collective action

Collective action for change does not happen overnight. It is a result of a growing critical awareness of a social or health problem and recognition of the need to come together and instigate change. The writings of Brazilian educator Paulo Freire (1970, 1973) can help us to understand why developing a critical consciousness is important to spark collective action and change, as well as how this is achieved.

To do this, Freire uses the example of didactic and top-down teaching, a pedagogical approach adopted in many parts of the world, to argue that such an approach to teaching assumes learners are passive beings in need of controlled knowledge, failing to foster critical thinking, and serves the purpose of keeping the rich and the elite in power and to further oppress the poor and powerless. Freire therefore calls for an alternative approach to teaching, one where learners and teachers engage in dialogue as equals, making the learners integral to the learning process, as opposed to objects. For Freire, education should be about creating safe social spaces for dialogue to occur, allowing people to share their life experiences and as a collective, and individually, develop ideas, new understandings, and ultimately a more critical awareness of self and other. Critical thinking, Freire (1973) argues, evolves over a series of stages, starting with 'intransitive thought'. At this stage people do not see it as within their power and control to instigate change and improve their life situation. If change does happen, this is likely to be explained by the influence of wider social structures, or even luck. The next stage towards more critical thinking pertains to 'semi-transitive' thought. Here people begin to see the connection between their actions and change to their lived realities, and experiment with various actions to instigate change. At this stage, however, they may still struggle to connect their social problems with the wider social structures and determinants that impact their lives. The final stage Freire refers to as 'critical transitivity'. At this stage people are experiencing an awakening of critical consciousness, or *conscientização* as Freire called it, and are able to critically engage with their life situation and see the connection between their social problems, or poor health, and the structural violence, oppression, and social inequalities that keep them in this condition. This will spark their interest to instigate change.

In summary, the change theory of this conceptual perspective is that creating social spaces for reflection and critical dialogue is a vehicle towards a more critical consciousness, where people become critically aware of their social situation as well as empowered, increasing the likelihood, and their interest, to translate this awareness into collective action and thereby instigate change.

One strength of this theoretical exposition is that it highlights the importance of seeing development as a process, involving a partnership between both those with more and less power. The theory can be used by health promoters to reflect on how they engage with people at a community level to build their critical awareness of health matters to instigate change. Photovoice, a health promotion tool rooted in Freire's conscientization theory, is described later in this chapter as one potential tool to facilitate community level change.

A limitation of the theory is that it fails to fully recognize the importance of 'awakened' people or communities to build partnerships with more resourceful actors such as health promoters. People and communities may, for example, be fully aware of the health implications of drinking water from a water hole also used by livestock, but do not have the resources and means to build a fencing system and water troughs, or money for transport to go and lobby for change. Critical awareness is a prerequisite for community level change, but we should not assume that this automatically translates into change and collective action.

Community participation

Although community participation more often occurs naturally and through indigenous social networks and groups – and from which much can be learnt – the focus here is on the role of health promoters in drawing on the concept of community participation to facilitate more health-enabling social environments. Community participation is a central tenet health promotion. It is widely accepted that only when externally facilitated health programmes recognize and draw on local structures and ways of life will they resonate with local needs, be relevant and contribute to changes in health-related behaviours and an effective community response to health. As a concept, community participation is a minefield, with its meaning always being contextual and partial, reflecting varying understandings and commitments to the term. Community participation can, for example, take different forms and reflect different degrees of community involvement. Peter Oakley (1991) distinguishes between three types of participation:

- *Participation as a free resource*: Community members may be invited to get involved in a project, implementing activities. This kind of participation is often marginal and primarily involves community members in order to tap into community resources (e.g. labour, land, knowledge, time). This kind of participation does not seek to empower or appropriate a health promotion initiative to local needs, but is used to meet externally designed programme goals and to use community members as a free resource. For example, unpaid community health workers trained by an external change agent to improve the hygiene and hand washing practices of community members in a rural community might spend hours trekking from household to household talking to them about their hand washing practices.
- *Participation as consultation*: In this type of participation, community members may be asked about their priorities, possible solutions to a local health need, as well as their level of involvement in the programme. The external change agent will, however, still retain control over the aim of the programme and the kind of activities that will be implemented. For example, a health promotion initiative looking to reduce HIV transmission among sex workers might consult sex workers about their sexual health needs and learn that they want improved condom access and sexual health education by peer educators. The external change agent might improve condom access, train peer educators, and have them facilitate sexual health education, but may decide to only improve condom access if that was the prearranged aim.
- *Participation as community control*: This level of participation allows community members to have complete control of the health initiative. For example, a sex workers' network may be mobilized as part of a health promotion initiative. But rather than having a set of prescribed project goals and activities imposed upon them, they conduct a needs assessment of their health needs, develop solutions, carry out activities, and evaluate progress. In other words, community members play an integral role in implementing the health promotion initiative, from start to finish.

While there is a role for all three levels of participation, depending on the context, community-level health promotion initiatives ought to strive for participation as community control. There are a number of reasons for this. Aside from appropriating and contextualizing a health promotion initiative, ensuring there is a good fit with local needs, community control of the planning and design of health promotion initiatives ensures community members are more likely to get involved and stay committed to the long-term goals of the initiative. Barriers to health can also be more easily identified and addressed, optimizing the impact of health promotion initiatives. But more importantly, participation as community control recognizes participation as a process as opposed to an activity used to achieve a single health outcome. Reflecting Freire's theory of *conscientization*, the process of community members conducting a needs assessment, gathering and analysing information about local health needs improves their consciousness, making it easier for them, as a community, to transform and negotiate new and more health-enabling norms and behaviours. Furthermore, the participatory process of community-led project cycles can be empowering, and ensures the participation and commitment of community members to the programme in the long term. Their experiences of taking an active role in the implementation of a programme can facilitate a sense of worthiness, enhance their internal locus of control and self-efficacy as well as a positive social orientation (Skovdal et al., 2011c). Participatory programmes can also improve individual and collective problem-solving abilities, improve social relationships and give them hope for the future. These are only some of the many social psychological outcomes that participatory processes may facilitate and represent protective processes that are of great value in enhancing the resilience of individuals and communities (Rutter, 1987).

In summary, the change theory of this conceptual perspective is that creating opportunities for community participation can, if done meaningfully and with community members taking an active and direct role in implementing a health promotion initiative, facilitate an educational process and dialogue that can help communities transform attitudes, norms, and actions that are health-damaging into more health-enhancing lifestyles. Community participation can also be empowering, and in the vein of *conscientization*, give people the chance to take control over different aspects of their lives, including their health.

A key strength of community participation as a conceptual tool in health promotion is that it is endorsed by global health policies, particularly in the wake of the Declaration of Alma Ata in 1977. As a result, community participation is widely recognized to be a key pillar in any health and development initiative, which makes it easier for practitioners at a community level to promote community participation for improved health.

A limitation of community participation is that the meanings of 'community' and 'participation' vary between people and over time. The boundaries of communities are fluid and are constantly shifting, and participation can range from being merely a free resource to encompass community control. Participatory community health promotion programmes can also easily be hijacked by more powerful individuals, both at local and global levels, to serve their own interests and undermine the participatory process (Cooke and Kothari, 2001). Another limitation pertains to the difficulty of measuring and evaluating community participation. The Spidergram, a tool developed by Susan Rifkin and colleagues to measure the participatory process, is described later in this chapter as one potential tool to facilitate and evaluate community level change.

Social capital

Social capital refers to the glue that brings people and different actors together for the common good. The term was popularized by Robert Putnam in the 1990s. He defines social capital as the community cohesion that results from 'networks, norms and social ties that facilitate coordination and cooperation for mutual benefit' (Putnam, 1995: 67). More specifically, communities with high levels of social capital are characterized by having a high number of active community organizations and networks, strong commitments to civic engagement or participation within these networks, as well as an ethics of care and reciprocal support, and a sense of solidarity and trust between community members. Although Putnam used the term to describe the socio-economic and political implications of declines in social capital, a growing body of evidence suggests that communities characterized by high levels of social capital are more likely to be healthy and engage in health-enhancing activities. As a result, a key aim of health promoters working at a community level is to facilitate the development of social capital.

Social capital theory builds on the two previous conceptual perspectives. In fact, conscientization and community participation contribute to the development of social capital, in so far as they seek to create a context where people can come together and take control over their health by transforming health-damaging behaviours and social identities. In the context of health promotion, and the previous discussion on health-enabling social environments, it is useful to unpack social capital and discuss the concept from three different perspectives: bonding, bridging, and linking social capital (Szreter and Woolcock, 2004).

Bonding social capital refers to the trust and quality of cooperative social relations that exist between members of a network or community, where members share similar characteristics. This could range from a little women's group made up of elderly widowed women who have come together to deal with hardship and the care and support of orphaned children, through to the collective response by a village or community to fight off tsetse flies and sleeping sickness. *Bridging* social capital, on the other hand, refers to horizontal relations of respect and empathy between people, groups or networks whose backgrounds are different, because of factors such as religious beliefs, viewpoints, age, ethnicity, sexuality, and social class. For example, in a low-resource and high HIV prevalent community, a church group and an AIDS support group might decide to come together and create a synergy to reduce HIV-related stigma in the community. *Linking* social capital refers to the bridging of relations of trust and respect between people, networks, and organizations whereby they interact vertically across power and authority structures. For example, a youth theatre group established to communicate HIV prevention messages may link up with a more resourceful non-governmental organization that can provide the group with the resources it requires to move around and reach a large number of people.

In summary, the change theory of social capital is that strengthening the connections between individuals, groups, and organizations (bonding, bridging, and linking social capital) equips community contexts with an asset that makes them stronger in times of hardship and which can be leveraged to maintain or improve health and well-being.

According to Szreter and Woolcock (2004), a strength of social capital theory is that it acknowledges the importance of recognizing the quality and quantity of social relations between individuals, groups, and organizations influencing health. The theory also encourages an emphasis on whether or not these social relationships are characterized by mutual respect or differentiated by social identities (horizontal bridges) and their access to power or authority (vertical links).

A limitation pertains to the controversy and criticism that surrounds the theory of social capital. Like community participation, concerns have been raised about the ambiguity of social capital and fears that social capital can be used to justify a withdrawal of government welfare services, with the explanation that communities with high levels of social capital have the power to fulfil this social welfare role (Labonte, 1999). Furthermore, social capital does not always carry with it positive health implications. A rural African community may, for example, avail support to the sick and elderly in many different ways and exhibit high levels of social capital for those who conform to the status quo of community life. While this is beneficial to the majority of community members, narrowly conscribed networks can simultaneously reject more stigmatized groups, such as men who have sex with men, leaving them extremely marginalized and vulnerable.

The asset model

Traditional health promotion models tend to focus on epidemiological risk factors, such as smoking, poor diet, and lack of exercise. In doing so, they take a deficit approach by focusing on gaps in services, information, and capacity. By contrast, the asset model looks at the resources of individuals and communities and how these can be harnessed to improve health and well-being. These resources or 'health assets' are defined as anything that maximizes opportunities for individuals and local communities to acquire, maintain, and sustain health and well-being (Ziglio et al., in press).

Health assets can include factors from across the range of the determinants of health, including genetic make-up, economic and social conditions, environmental conditions, health behaviour, and use of health and other services. Research by the WHO European Office for Investment in Health and Development (Harrison et al., 2004) identified key health assets to include family and friendship networks, inter-generational solidarity, community cohesion, environmental resources necessary for promoting physical, mental and social health, employment security and opportunities for voluntary service, affinity groups (such as mutual aid), religious tolerance and har-mony, life-long learning, safe and pleasant housing, political democracy and participation opportunities, social justice and enhancing equity. The assets for health that are amen-able to action are often located at the community level, so an asset-based approach is closely aligned with community development.

Three concepts are central to the asset model. First, the concept of salutogenesis, introduced by Aaron Antonovsky in 1979, focuses attention on health generation rather than a pathogenesis focus on disease prevention. Salutogenesis emphasizes the success rather than the failure of individuals by exploring why some people prosper and others fall ill in similar situations (Antonovsky, 1979, 1987, 1996). Second, the asset model sees resilience as a protective factor for both individuals and communities to thrive, even in the face of difficult circumstances. Third, the model sees the concept of social capital, as discussed above, as key to creating strong supportive networks for health, well-being, and development.

The asset model suggests that individuals and communities can develop health assets at various stages of life and can use these to offset risks that they face as they age and at critical moments during their life, such as early childhood, entering the labour mar-ket, parenthood, sickness, job loss, and old age. The model argues there are core sets of assets, linked to the concepts of salutogenesis, resilience and social capital, that are key for the successful transition through these stages. It is also recognized that particular assets will impact in different ways depending on individual circumstances. The model suggests understanding which asset or combination of assets is most important at key transitional stages can help develop more effective programmes to improve well-being and health.

Ziglio et al. (in press) have highlighted the following key features of the asset model:

1 It fosters a systematic approach to developing a coherent evidence base for positive approaches to health and development following the principles of evidence-based public health.
2 It emphasizes those health-promoting and protective factors ('health assets') that can support the creation of the conditions required for acquiring, maintaining, and sustaining health and well-being.
3 It highlights the potential for a set of key theories, methods, and actions that can be employed to develop asset-based policy, research, and practice.
4 It recognizes that many of the key assets for health creation lie within the social context of people's lives and therefore offers the opportunity of contributing to the health inequity agenda.
5 It assumes that to maximize the opportunity for identifying health assets, individuals and communities need to be involved in all aspects of the health development process.
6 It is about working with what communities already have, rather than assuming there is nothing there to start with. In this way, it encourages individuals and communities to be active partners in the process, rather than passive recipients.

7 It emphasizes the importance of a life course approach to the promotion of health, recognizing that different assets may be more or less important at key life stages.

8 It is does not preclude the need to employ the well-developed deficit approaches to health, but offers a model that may work synergistically to sustain health and minimize inequities.

9 It ensures existing resources at the individual, community or organizational level are taken into account.

10 It looks to the individual with their formal and informal associations within the community to create solutions and mobilize capacity to achieve better health.

There are many overlaps between the four conceptual perspectives discussed above. They all build on each other and are rooted in a common recognition of the need to draw on local strengths in creating health-enabling social environments and promote a development process where gradients of power and authority are more aligned and characterized by mutual respect.

Activity 6.3

In this activity, you will consider the role of communities in theories of change. What changes would you like to make to the theory of change you developed in the previous activity to incorporate the four conceptual perspectives you have just been introduced to?

Feedback

Your theory of change should not only reflect an understanding of one or a hybrid of the conceptual frameworks explained above, but also a broader recognition of the steps in the process of change and your role as a change agent.

Tools to facilitate community level change

The conceptual perspectives discussed above highlight the importance of community engagement and empowerment in guiding change at a community level for improved health. There are a number of different participatory learning and action tools that can be employed to facilitate such a process. Participatory learning and action tools seek to visually generate different forms of information, which can then be used by community members to reflect, engage in dialogue, and make collective and democratic decisions. Maps, diagrams, pictures, and charts can all be used by community members to visually represent information gathered from their local context, while ranking and scoring tools can be used to facilitate decision-making processes in a democratic manner.

The following two examples illustrate techniques that can be used to apply the theories of change described above in practice. Additional detailed examples of many of the tools that can be used to engage communities are provided in Rifkin and Pridmore's book *Partners in Planning: Information, Participation and Empowerment* (2001) and *Tools Together Now: 100 Participatory Tools to Mobilise Communities for HIV/AIDS* (2006), available on the worldwide web from the International HIV/AIDS Alliance.

Example 1: Photovoice

Photovoice is a technique that enables community members to visually represent aspects of community life through picture taking. The pictures can be used to reflect on the community's strengths and problems as well as a means to share this information with fellow community members, health service providers or policy actors (Wang et al., 1998). In doing so, Photovoice can act as a bridge between local realities and expert priorities, sharpening policy and practice for a better fit with local needs. Photovoice can also cultivate critical dialogue and reflection at a local level, which can instigate cognitive-emotional reactions leading to individual or collective change. In essence, Photovoice stimulates a sharing of information, across languages, literacy and power hierarchies in the hope that this can lead to more aligned knowledge systems and priorities, appropriating community responses, programmes, and policies for health.

Photovoice is a flexible tool and needs to be adapted to each context. In the field of health promotion, Photovoice is often used as an assessment tool, both in the planning and evaluation of health promotion initiatives. The implementation process can take multiple forms. Below is an outline of key steps (adapted from Wang, 2006) that can help you get started.

Photovoice implementation steps

1. Recruit a group of Photovoice participants
- 7–15 people is an ideal size (more have often been used).
- You can recruit through educational establishments, churches, profit and non-profit organizations.
- If you recruit different groups (e.g. youth/adults, employers/employees, men/women), you can gain comparative perspectives.

2. Introduce the Photovoice methodology to participants and discuss the use of cameras, power, and ethics
- What is an acceptable way to approach someone to take their picture?
- Can you take pictures of other people without their knowledge?
- When would you not want to have your picture taken?
- To whom might you wish to give the photographs?
- And what might be the implications?

3. Obtain informed consent
- Place emphasis on the safety, authority, and responsibility of using a camera.
- Consider the vulnerability of the photographer; include a statement of potential risks.
- Clarify the voluntary nature of their participation, and the freedom to withdraw at any time without giving a reason.
- No photographs identifying specific individuals should be released without separate written consent.
- Obtain informed consent from parents or guardians for all minors.

4. Pose initial themes for taking pictures
- Participants can generate, or be given, specific open-ended questions that will guide the taking of pictures.

5. Distribute cameras to participants
- Decide on using disposable or digital cameras and practise using them.
- Agree on a time for participants to return the cameras/images for developing/print.

- 1–5 weeks per roll of film is recommended before meeting up again (this process has on occasions been repeated for up to 12 months).
- Agree on a time for participants to discuss the photographs/write reflections.

6. Discuss photographs and identify themes
- Discuss photographs, or a selection based on a prescribed criterion or based on what the participants find most significant or like the most.
- Facilitate a group discussion, asking them to describe the photographs, explain what is happening on the photographs, their reasons for taking the photographs, the significance of the photographs, and lessons learnt from the photographs.
- Photographs can also be reflected upon in writing, prompted by open-ended questions.
- Participants identify key themes emerging from their photographs and reflections.

7. Dissemination
- Facilitate the creation of posters/power point presentations depicting key takeaway messages using the photographs and voices of the participants and exhibit them in a public space.

Example 2: Spidergrams

A Spidergram is a web-like diagram that can be used by community members themselves to evaluate community health competence or community participation (Rifkin and Pridmore, 2001; Draper et al., 2010). Community members can come together to discuss a health issue and decide to assess their competence, or preparedness, in this area, marking themselves on a scale of 1 (poor) to 5 (excellent) on various categories. Spidergrams can be drawn up before a health promotion programme, giving community members a chance to reflect on what changes need to be made, and at the end of the programme to see if the community's level of health competence has changed during the course of the programme. This exercise can give community members an insight into some of their strengths and weaknesses in working towards a more health-enabling social environment as well as clarify their role in the response towards improved health.

The Spidergram depicted in Figure 6.3 shows a community assessing their competence in relation to children caring for sick parents. The example shows a dotted (time 1) and a solid (time 2) spider web, depicting change in community health competence from one moment in time to another (e.g. before and after a health promotion initiative). The Spidergram in this example incorporates eight key areas important to community-level health promotion, reflecting the material presented in this chapter. However, the Spidergram could have fewer arms and be used to assess participation in areas such as leadership, organization, resource mobilization, management, and needs assessment.

Activity 6.4

In this activity, you will consider the practical issues involved in engaging communities to plan a health promotion intervention using Photovoice. Think of a local context familiar to you and a health issue that this community is battling with. You would like to make the wider community more critically aware of this health issue, as well ensure

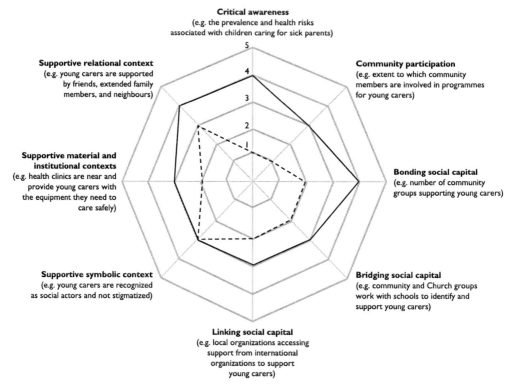

Figure 6.3 Spidergram for community health competence

Source: Adapted from Draper et al. (2010)

that the local health department is aware of the information you will gather in the process. You decide to use Photovoice. Develop a plan detailing your implementation steps.

Feedback

There are a number of questions you might consider in developing your plan. These include:

- What are your broader goals and objectives?
- Where will funding come from?
- What community leaders should be involved?
- Who are you targeting – policy-makers, community leaders?
- How many will be involved in the Photovoice exercise?
- Will they be working individually or in groups?
- What is their involvement in the planning of your Photovoice project?
- How (content) will you train them on the methodology? Use of cameras? Ethics?
- What informed consent measures must be in place?

- What is guiding their photography? Think of questions they can answer through photography
- How long will the project last?
- How many photos/rolls of film do you expect them to take?
- How often do you meet to discuss photographs?
- In what fora will you be discussing the pictures – group discussions, in writing?
- How do you intend to reach the target audience?
- How will the findings be disseminated?

Remember, Photovoice is flexible and there is no set guideline on how to implement a Photovoice project. Use your creativity and local knowledge to develop a project that has the greatest chance of instigating change for improved health.

Skills and attitudes of health promoters at a community level

Health promotion at a community level is not apolitical and should not be reduced to tasks, tools, and technical solutions. Health promoters work within wider societal structures that are characterized by power, resources, and dominant health technologies. Community health promoters are therefore often given the very difficult task of serving as intermediaries between health professionals and people at a community level, bridging global health technologies and local responses to improved health. The values of health promoters and how they approach their role and work with communities therefore matter tremendously. Developing partnerships that transcend power hierarchies, conflicting values and knowledge systems, and successfully working together to promote the health and well-being of marginalized people, requires good interpersonal and cross-cultural communication skills. It is very easy for community health promoters to succumb to the production of expert and technical solutions, particularly if a genuine and deep-seated commitment to community development, empowerment, principles of social justice, and the need for community-defined problems and solutions is lacking. Community health promotion is arguably not for everyone. It is the role of the health promoter to recognize his or her commitment to community work and to:

- be reflective of power hierarchies and structures, both within communities and between local and global actors
- recognize, respect, and be committed to the principles of community participation and social justice
- be a good facilitator, develop skills to be a good listener, be positive, respectful, and open to new ideas.

Summary

In this chapter, you have learnt how theories can help you conceive and plan health promotion programmes at a community level. More specifically, you have learnt about the role of critical awareness, participation, and social capital in creating health-enabling social environments that empower people to take control over their own health, and the health of others. The chapter has also highlighted that health promotion practice at the community level needs to be nested within a context, ranging from the wider social influences that enable and limit community level health responses to the values and interpersonal skills of health promoters. Only by taking this holistic view will we be able to create the necessary conditions for health through community empowerment and participation.

References

Antonovsky, A. (1979) *Health, Stress and Coping.* San Francisco, CA: Jossey-Bass.

Antonovsky, A. (1987) *Unravelling the Mystery of Health: How People Manage Stress and Stay Well.* San Francisco, CA: Jossey-Bass.

Antonovsky, A. (1996) The salutogenic model as a theory to guide health promotion, *Health Promotion International*, 11(1): 11–18.

Bronfenbrenner, U. (1979) *The Ecology of Human Development: Experiments by Nature and Design.* Cambridge, MA: Harvard University Press.

Campbell, C. (2001) Social capital and health: contextualising health promotion within local community networks, in T. Schuller, S.R. Baron and J. Field (eds.) *Social Capital: Critical Perspectives.* Oxford: Oxford University Press.

Campbell, C. and Cornish, F. (2010) Towards a 'fourth generation' of approaches to HIV/AIDS management: creating contexts for effective community mobilisation, *AIDS Care*, 22(suppl. 2): 1569–79.

Campbell, C., Scott, K., Nhamo, M., Nyamukapa, C., Madanhire, C., Skovdal, M. et al. (in press) Social capital and HIV competent communities: the role of community groups in managing HIV/AIDS in rural Zimbabwe, *AIDS Care*.

Cooke, B. and Kothari, U. (2001) *Participation, the New Tyranny?* London: Zed Books.

Draper, A.K., Hewitt, G. and Rifkin, S. (2010) Chasing the dragon: developing indicators for the assessment of community participation in health programmes, *Social Science and Medicine*, 71(6): 1102–9.

Freire, P. (1970) *Pedagogy of the Oppressed.* London: Penguin.

Freire, P. (1973) *Education for Critical Consciousness.* New York: Seabury Press.

Gregson, S., Nyamukapa, C., Schumacher, C., Magutshwa-Zitha, S., Skovdal, M., Yekeye, R. et al. (in press) Evidence for a contribution of the community response to HIV decline in eastern Zimbabwe, *AIDS Care*.

Harrison, D., Ziglio, E., Levin, L. and Morgan, A. (2004) *Assets for Health and Development: Developing a Conceptual Framework.* Venice: European Office for Investment for Health and Development, World Health Organization.

Labonte, R. (1999) Social capital and community development: practitioner emptor, *Australian and New Zealand Journal of Public Health*, 23(4): 430–433.

Oakley, P. (1991) *Projects with People: The Practice of Participation in Rural Development.* Geneva: International Labour Office.

Putnam, R. (1995) Bowling alone: America's declining social capital, *Journal of Democracy*, 6(1): 65–78.

Rifkin, S. and Pridmore, P. (2001) *Partners in Planning: Information, Participation and Empowerment.* London: TALC/Macmillan Education.

Rutter, M. (1987) Psychosocial resilience and protective factors, *American Journal of Orthopsychiatry*, 57: 316–31.

Skovdal, M., Campbell, C., Madanhire, C., Mupambireyi, Z., Nyamukapa, C. and Gregson, S. (2011a) Masculinity as a barrier to men's use of HIV services in Zimbabwe, *Globalisation and Health*, 7: 13.

Skovdal, M., Campbell, C., Nhongo, K., Nyamukapa, C. and Gregson, S. (2011b) Contextual and psychosocial influences on antiretroviral therapy adherence in rural Zimbabwe: towards a systematic framework for programme planners, *International Journal of Health Planning and Management*, 26(3): 296–318.

Skovdal, M., Mwasiaji, W., Webale, A. and Tomkins, A. (2011c) Building orphan competent communities: experiences from a community-based capital cash transfer initiative in Kenya, *Health Policy and Planning*, 26(3): 233–41.

Stokols, D. (1996) Translating social ecological theory into guidelines for community health promotion, *American Journal of Health Promotion*, 10(4): 282–98.

Szreter, S. and Woolcock, M. (2004) Health by association? Social capital, social theory, and the political economy of public health, *International Journal of Epidemiology*, 33(4): 650–67.

Wang, C. (2006) Youth participation in Photovoice as a strategy for community change, in B.N. Checkoway and L.M. Gutiérrez (eds.) *Youth Participation and Community Change*. Binghamton, NY: Haworth Press.

Wang, C.C., Yi, W.K., Tao, Z.W. and Carovano, K. (1998) Photovoice as a participatory health promotion strategy, *Health Promotion International*, 13(1): 75–86.

Ziglio, E., Morgan, A., Burns, H., Hernan, M. and Barker, R. (in press) *Maximising Health Potential for 2020: The Asset Model for Health and Development*. Venice: European Office for Investment for Health and Development, World Health Organization.

Further reading

International HIV/AIDS Alliance (2006) *Tools Together Now: 100 Participatory Tools to Mobilise Communities for HIV/AIDS*. Available at: http://www.aidsalliance.org/includes/Publication/Tools_Together_Now_2009.pdf.

Morgan, A. and Ziglio, E. (2007) Revitalising the evidence base for public health: an assets model, *Promotion and Education*, 14(2 suppl.): 17–22.

Morgan, A., Davies, M. and Ziglio, E. (2010) *Health Assets in a Global Context: Theory, Methods, Action*. New York: Springer.

Nishtar, S. (ed.) (2007) Community health promotion: creating the necessary conditions for health through community empowerment and participation, *Promotion and Education*, XIV(2): 61–134.

Rifkin, S. and Pridmore, P. (2001) *Partners in Planning: Information, Participation and Empowerment*. London: TALC/Macmillan Education.

7 | The determinants of health

Antony Morgan and Liza Cragg

Overview

In this chapter, you will learn about the range of factors that have an impact on the ability of individuals, communities, and societies to develop and maintain good health and well-being. The chapter highlights the importance of the social determinants of health, explores conceptual models and evidence for these determinants, discusses global policy developments, and summarizes the implications for health promotion practice.

Learning objectives

After reading this chapter, you will be able to:

- describe the major determinants of health
- understand different conceptual models that describe these determinants
- understand the role of the social determinants of health in causing health inequities
- understand the implications of the determinants of health for health promotion practice

Key terms

Determinants of health: The range of factors that combine together to affect the health of individuals.

Inequalities in health: Differences in health status between different populations and groups.

Social determinants of health: The social, economic, and environmental factors that impact on health behaviours and determine the health status of individuals or populations.

Social inequities: Differences in opportunity for different population sub-groups.

Socio-economic status: An individual's place in the social hierarchy according to their level of income, education, occupation, and/or where they live.

What determines health?

Health and well-being are influenced by a range of factors. These include individual characteristics and behaviour, the physical environment, and the social and economic conditions. Some of these factors can be influenced by an individual's action, such as lifestyle. Others, such as genetic make up and gender, cannot be changed. These factors are often described as the 'determinants of health'. While some of these have obvious and direct impacts on health, such as the provision of health care services, others, such as employment and education, influence health in more indirect but very significant ways. The social and economic circumstances that impact upon health and well-being – the conditions in which we are born, grow up, live, work, and age – are termed the 'social determinants of health'. These factors have been described as the causes of illness. For example, while smoking causes illnesses such as coronary heart disease and lung cancer, whether an individual is likely to start smoking or stop smoking is heavily influenced by social, economic, and environmental factors.

Activity 7.1

This activity encourages you to reflect on factors that influence health. Think about the following questions:

- What does it mean to be healthy?
- What factors help people to be healthy and stay healthy?
- What are some of the causes of ill health?
- What are the causes of these causes?

Feedback

In answer to the first question, you might have concluded that being healthy means not being ill or in pain. But health is more than this. The World Health Organization's definition of health is 'not merely the absence of disease but a state of complete physical, mental and social well-being'. In response to the second question, your answer may have included factors such as having access to healthy food, clean water, health care, housing, and sanitation. In addition to these basic needs, you might have included lifestyle factors such as taking exercise, getting rest, being relaxed, and free from stress. Moving on to the third question, lacking these basic needs causes ill health but ill health can also be caused by lifestyle factors, such as unhealthy eating, smoking or lack of exercise. In response to the final question, your answer should reflect that the causes of the causes of ill health also include lack of income to secure basic needs, poor education, unemployment or hazardous working conditions, inadequate access to health care or poor quality health care, poor quality physical environment, pollution, and lack of support networks.

Conceptualizing the determinants of health

The Lalonde Report (1974) was one of the first documents to propose a framework to describe the determinants of health. It introduced the Health Field Concept, which

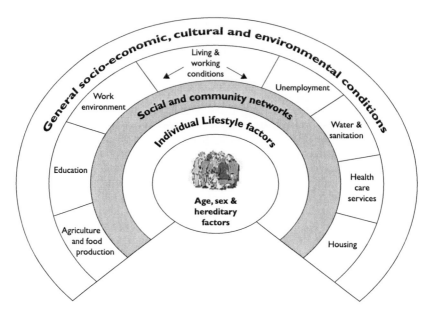

Figure 7.1 The policy rainbow. From Dahlgren, G., Whitehead, M. (1991) Policies and strategies to promote social equity in health (mimeo). Reproduced by permission of Institute for Future Studies, Stockholm.

described four categories of influences on health. These categories, which were identified by analysing the causes and underlying factors of sickness and death in Canada, were: human biology, environment, lifestyle, and health care organization. Activity 7.2 explores the Lalonde Report in more detail.

Since the Lalonde Report, a number of other models that attempt to identify the determinants of health and the pathways through which they operate have been developed. One such model that has been used frequently in international and national policy documents is Dahlgren and Whitehead's (1991) 'policy rainbow'. This describes the layers of influence on an individual's potential for health (Figure 7.1). These are made up of factors which are fixed (such as age, sex, and genetics) and factors which are potentially modifiable, expressed as a series of layers of influence, including individual lifestyle factors, social and community networks, and general socio-economic, cultural, and environmental conditions.

The model of Dahlgren and Whitehead provided a useful framework for exploring the mechanisms by which these factors, or determinants, influence health, their relative importance, and how to influence them to improve health and well-being.

Over the last few decades, researchers have generated a growing body of evidence that demonstrates how a wide range of determinants impact on health and well-being. Examples include:

- Marmot et al. (1978) have demonstrated gradients in mortality across grades of employment among English civil servants.
- Bartley et al. (1994) have shown that children and adolescents living in poorer quality housing are more likely to have been of low birth weight.

- Townsend et al. (1988) have shown that material deprivation (e.g. overcrowding, housing tenure, unemployment) is a predictor of mortality and limiting long-term illness.
- Barker (1998) has shown that the *in utero* experience is linked to the risk of developing diseases later in life.
- Graham (2001) has demonstrated the cumulative effect of social disadvantage over the life course and the contribution of poor early life circumstances.
- McGinnis et al. (2002) have demonstrated the relative impact that various health determinants make on mortality in the USA: 30 per cent due to genetic predispositions, 15 per cent due to social circumstances, 5 per cent due to environmental exposures, 40 per cent due to behavioural patterns, and 10 per cent due to shortfalls in health care.

Activity 7.2

In this activity, you will explore how one model, the Health Field Concept, categorizes the determinants of health and reflect on the benefits and limitations of this approach. Read the following extracts from the Lalonde Report (1974). Once you have done this, answer the questions that follow.

The Health Field Concept

A basic problem in analysing the health field has been the absence of an agreed conceptual framework for sub-dividing it into its principal elements. Without such a framework, it has been difficult to communicate properly or to break up the field into manageable segments, amenable to analysis and evaluation. It was felt keenly that there was a need to organize the thousands of pieces into an orderly pattern that was both intellectually acceptable and sufficiently simple to permit the quick location, in the pattern, of almost any idea, problem or activity related to health: a sort of map of the health territory.

Such a Health Field Concept was developed during the preparation of this paper. It envisages that the health field can be broken up into four broad elements: HUMAN BIOLOGY, ENVIRONMENT, LIFESTYLE and HEALTH CARE ORGANIZATION. These four elements were identified through an examination of the causes and underlying factors of sickness and death in Canada and from an assessment of the parts these elements play in affecting the level of health in Canada.

Human Biology

The HUMAN BIOLOGY element includes all those aspects of health, both physical and mental, which are developed within the human body as a consequence of the basic biology of man and the organic make-up of the individual. This element includes the genetic inheritance of the individual, the processes of maturation and aging, and the body's many complex internal systems, such as skeletal, nervous, muscular, cardiovascular, endocrine, digestive and so on. As the human body is such a complicated organism, the health implications of human biology are numerous, varied and serious and the things that can go wrong with it are legion. Health problems originating from human biology are causing untold miseries and costing billions of dollars in treatment services.

Environment

The ENVIRONMENT category includes all those matters related to health which are external to the human body and over which the individual has little or no control. Individuals cannot, by themselves, ensure that foods, drugs, cosmetics, devices, water supply, etc. are safe and uncontaminated; that the health hazards of air, water and noise pollution are controlled; that the spread of communicable diseases is prevented; that effective garbage and sewage disposal is carried out; and that the social environment, including the rapid changes in it, do not have harmful effects on health.

Lifestyle

The LIFESTYLE category, in the Health Field Concept, consists of the aggregation of decisions by individuals which affect their health and over which they more or less have control ... Personal decisions and habits that are bad, from a health point of view, create self-imposed risks. When those risks result in illness or death, the victim's lifestyle can be said to have contributed to, or caused, this.

Health Care Organization

The fourth category in the concept is HEALTH CARE ORGANIZATION, which consists of the quantity, quality, arrangement, nature and relationships of people and resources in the provision of health care ... Until now most of society's efforts to improve health, and the bulk of direct health expenditures, have been focused on HEALTH CARE ORGANIZATION. Yet, when we identify the present main causes of sickness and death in Canada, we find that they are rooted in the other three elements of the Concept: HUMAN BIOLOGY, ENVIRONMENT and LIFESTYLE. It is apparent, therefore, that vast sums are being spent treating diseases that could have been prevented in the first place. Greater attention to the first three conceptual elements is needed if we are to continue to reduce disability and early death.

Characteristics of the Health Field Concept

The HEALTH FIELD CONCEPT has many characteristics which make it a powerful tool for analysing health problems, determining the health needs of Canadians and choosing the means by which those needs can be met.

One of the evident consequences of the Health Field Concept has been to raise HUMAN BIOLOGY, ENVIRONMENT and LIFESTYLE to a level of categorical importance, equal to that of HEALTH CARE ORGANIZATION. This, in itself, is a radical step in view of the clear pre-eminence that HEALTH CARE ORGANIZATION has had in past concepts of the health field.

A second attribute of the Concept is that it is comprehensive. Any health problem can be traced to one, or a combination, of the four elements. This comprehensiveness is important because it ensures that all aspects of health will be given due consideration and that all who contribute to health, individually and collectively – patient, physician, scientist and government – are aware of their roles and their influence on the level of health.

A third feature is that the Concept permits a system of analysis by which any question can be examined under the four elements in order to assess their relative significance and interaction. For example, the underlying causes of death from traffic accidents can be found to be due mainly to risks taken by individuals, with lesser importance given to the design of cars and roads, and to the availability of emergency treatment. Human biology has little or no significance in this area. In order of importance, therefore, LIFESTYLE, ENVIRONMENT and HEALTH CARE ORGANIZATION contribute to traffic deaths in the proportions of something like 75%, 20% and 5% respectively. This analysis permits programme planners to focus their attention on the most important contributing factors. Similar assessments of the relative importance of contributing factors can be made for many other health problems.

A fourth feature of the Concept is that it permits a further sub-division of factors. Again, for traffic deaths in the Lifestyle category, the risks taken by individuals can be classed under impaired driving, carelessness, failure to wear seat-belts and speeding. In many ways the Concept thus provides a road map which shows the most direct links between health problems, and their underlying causes, and the relative importance of various contributing factors.

Finally, the Health Field Concept provides a new perspective on health, a perspective which frees creative minds for the recognition and exploration of hitherto neglected fields. The importance for their own health of the behaviour and habits of individual Canadians is an example of the kind of conclusion that is obtainable by using the Health Field Concept as an analytical tool.

One of the main problems in improving the health of Canadians is that the essential power to do so is widely dispersed among individual citizens, governments, health professions and institutions. This fragmentation of responsibility has sometimes led to imbalanced approaches, with each participant in the health field pursuing solutions only within his area of interest. Under the Health Field Concept, the fragments are brought together into a unified whole which permits everyone to see the importance of all factors, including those which are the responsibility of others.

This unified view of the health field may well turn out to be one of the Concept's main contributions to progress in improving the level of health.

Issues arising from the use of the Health Field Concept

The Concept was designed with two aims in view: to provide a greater understanding of what contributes to sickness and death, and to facilitate the identification of courses of action that might be taken to improve health. The Concept is *not* an organizational framework for structuring programmes and activities to one or another of the four elements of the Concept and would be contrary to reality and would perpetuate the present fragmentary approach to solving health problems. For example, the problem of drug abuse needs attention by researchers in human biology, by behavioural scientists, by those who administer drug laws and by those who provide personal health care. Contributions are necessary from all of these and it would be a misuse of the Health Field Concept to exploit it as a basis for capturing all aspects of a problem for one particular unit of organization, or interest group ...

[Another] issue, more theoretical, was whether or not it was possible to divide external influences on health between the environment, about which the individual can do little, and lifestyle, in which he can make choices. Particularly cogent were arguments that personal choices were dictated by environmental factors, such as the peer-group pressures to start smoking cigarettes during the teens. Further, it was argued that some bad personal habits were so ingrained as to constitute addictions which, by definition, no longer permitted a choice by a simple act of will. Smoking, alcohol abuse and drug abuse were some of the lifestyle problems referred to in this vein. The fact that there is some truth in both hypotheses, i.e. that environment affects lifestyle and that some personal habits are addictive, requires a philosophical and moral response, rather than a purely intellectual one. This response is that if we simply give up on individuals whose lifestyles create excessive risks to their health, we will be abandoning those who could have changed, and will be perpetuating the very environment which influenced them adversely in the first place. In short, the deterministic view must be put aside in favour of faith in the power of free will, hobbled as this power may be at times by environment and addiction.

One point on which no quarter can be given is that difficulties in categorizing the contributing factors to a given health problem are no excuse for putting the problem aside. The problem does not disappear because of difficulties in fitting it nicely into a conceptual framework. Another issue is whether or not the Concept will be used to carry too much of an analytical workload, by demanding that it serve both to identify requirements for health and to determine the mechanisms for meeting them. Although the Concept will help bring out the problems and their causes and even point to the avenues by which they can be solved, it cannot determine the precise steps that are needed to implement programmes. Decisions as to programmes are affected by so many other considerations that they will require the analysis of many practical factors outside the Concept proper.

The ultimate philosophical issue raised by the Concept is whether, and to what extent, government can get into the business of modifying human behaviour, even if it does so to improve health. The marketing of social change is a new field which applies the marketing techniques of the business world to getting people to change their behaviour, i.e. eating habits, exercise habits, smoking habits, driving habits, etc. It is argued by some that proficiency in social marketing would inevitably lead governments into all kinds of undesirable thought control and propaganda. The dangers of governmental proficiency in social marketing are recognized, but so are the evident abuses resulting from all other kinds of marketing. If the siren song of coloured television, for example, is creating an indolent and passive use of leisure time, has the government not the duty to counteract its effects by marketing programmes aimed at promoting physical recreation? As previously mentioned, in Canada some 76% of the population over age 13 devotes less than one hour a week to participation in sports, while 84% of the same population spends four or more hours weekly watching television. This kind of imbalance extends to the amount of money being spent by the private sector on marketing products and services, some of which, if abused, contribute to sickness and death. One must inevitably conclude that society, through government, owes it to itself to develop protective marketing techniques to counteract those abuses.

Finally, some have questioned whether an increased emphasis on human biology, environment and lifestyle will not lead to a diminution of attention to the system of personal health care. This issue is raised particularly by those whose activities are centred on the health care organization. On this issue it can be said, that Canadians would not tolerate a reduction in personal health care and are in fact pushing very hard to make services more accessible and more comprehensive ...

More important, if the incidence of sickness can be reduced by prevention then the cost of present services will go down, or at least the rate of increase will diminish. This will make money available to extend health insurance to more and more services and to provide needed facilities, such as ambulatory care centres and extended care institutions. To a considerable extent, therefore, the increased availability of health care services to Canadians depends upon the success that can be achieved in preventing illness through measures taken in human biology, environment and lifestyle.

(Extracts from *the Lalonde report on the field health concept.* Lalonde, M., (1974) *A New Perspective on the Health of Canadians: A Working Document.* Marc Lalonde, Minister of National Health and Welfare, 1974, c1981. Reproduced by permission of the Minister of Health of Canada, 2013.

- What does the Lalonde Report propose are the main influences on health status and their relative importance?
- What does the report suggest are the main benefits of the Health Field Concept approach?
- What does the report say are the limitations of this approach? Can you think of any others?

Feedback

1 The main influences on health status are: human biology, environment, lifestyle, and health care organization. The relative importance of each of these depends on the health issue concerned. For example, congenital anomalies will largely be due to human biology and the environment, whereas coronary heart disease will be determined by all four categories.

2 The Report proposes the main benefits of the approach are as follows: it gives environment, biology, and lifestyle the same importance as health care organization in understanding health; it is comprehensive and, therefore, allows everyone involved in health to play a role, not just doctors; it provides a framework for analysis so programme planners can focus on relevant factors; it reduces fragmentation of responsibility between different actors; and improving prevention can reduce the costs, or the rate of increase in costs, of treatment services. These savings can then be re-invested in health.

3 The Report suggests the limitations of the approach are as follows: it should not be seen as an organizational tool for structuring programmes, as this could lead to further fragmentation; it cannot determine how to implement programmes; and it could be used to justify reductions in health care expenditure. You might also have observed that some of the analysis is dependent on norms that are now outdated. For example, most people working to prevent road accidents would now emphasize the importance of the environment over the lifestyle factors that Lalonde focused on.

The social determinants and inequalities in health

Research on how the social determinants have impacted health over the last 30 years has documented how health is socially patterned (Townsend et al., 1988; Harris et al., 1999). That is, while health status is influenced by individual characteristics and behaviour, it continues to be significantly determined by the different social, economic, and environmental circumstances of individuals and populations. In other words, people living in different socio-economic environments face different risks of ill health and death.

In general, the least affluent have much poorer health than the most affluent. Furthermore, it is notable that disease prevalence, life expectancy, behavioural risk factors, and general well-being indicate there is a 'social gradient' whereby there is a linear increase in ill health and mortality with decreasing socio-economic status (Marmot, 2004).

Inequalities in the social determinants of health are not the same as health inequalities. However, they are an important cause of health inequalities. Health inequalities that are preventable because they are caused by unequal access to the social determinants of health are often referred to as 'inequities in health' (CSDH, 2008). Health inequalities and the social gradient of health are discussed in more detail in Chapter 8.

The Commission on Social Determinants of Health

In response to growing concern globally about inequities in health between and within countries, the World Health Organization (WHO) set up the Commission on Social Determinants of Health (CSDH) in 2005. The CSDH was 'to marshal the evidence on what can be done to promote health equity, and to foster a global movement to achieve it' (CSDH, 2008: 3). The final report of the CSDH was published in 2008 (CSDH, 2008).

The CSDH took a holistic view of the determinants of health, which it defined as 'structural determinants and conditions of daily life' (CSDH, 2008: 1). In doing so, it recognized that 'by their nature many of the social determinants considered by the Commission are relatively distant, spatially and temporally, from individuals and health experience. This is challenging, both conceptually and empirically, when trying to attribute causality and demonstrate effectiveness of action on health equity' (CSDH, 2008: 42). The CSDH adopted a conceptual framework to describe how these determinants interact with each other to influence health and health inequities. This framework suggests that intervention for change needs to take action on the circumstances of daily life and the structural drivers. The framework is shown in Figure 7.2.

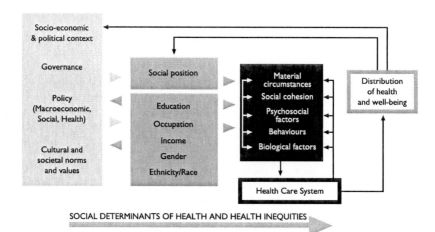

Figure 7.2 WHO Commission on the Social Determinants of Health Conceptual Framework. Reproduced by permission of the World Health Organization.

Given the wide range of issues covered in this holistic approach to the social determinants of health, the CSDH focused its work on those issues with a strong coherence
in the global evidence base and those with a strong plausible relationship with health
inequities but where evidence was still lacking on what could be done to effect change.
Using these criteria, the CSDH selected the following nine themes to explore in detail:

1 Early child development
2 Employment conditions
3 Urban settings
4 Social exclusion
5 Women and gender equity
6 Globalization
7 Health systems
8 Priority public health conditions
9 Measurement and evidence.

Based on its findings on these nine themes, the CSDH report proposes three principles for action, each supported by evidence and detailed recommendations: first,
improve daily living conditions; second, tackle the inequitable distribution of power,
money, and resources; and third, measure and understand the problem and assess the
impact of action.

Improve daily living conditions

This first principle is based on evidence that conditions of early childhood and school-
ing, employment and working conditions, and the quality of the natural and built environment in which people reside all impact on health outcomes. In particular, different
groups have different experiences of material conditions, psychosocial support, and
behavioural options, which make them more or less vulnerable to poor health.
Furthermore, socio-economic status results in differential access to and utilization of
health care, which causes the inequitable promotion of health and well-being, disease
prevention, and illness recovery and survival.

This principle for action reflects the CSDH's conclusion that experiences in early
childhood (defined as prenatal development to 8 years of age), and in early and later
education, lay the critical foundations for the entire life course. Consequently, it proposes a comprehensive approach to early life is needed, building on existing child survival programmes and extending interventions in early life to include social/emotional
and language/cognitive development. It recognizes evidence of the importance of
where people live in determining their health, including the role of urbanization in
reshaping population health problems, particularly among the urban poor, towards
non-communicable diseases, accidental and violent injuries, and deaths and impact from
ecological disaster. For example, in Nairobi, where 60% of the city's population lives in
slums, child mortality in the slums is 2.5 times greater than that in other areas of the
city (CSDH, 2008: 60). This principle also reflects the importance of work and employment conditions to health and well-being. The CSDH cites extensive evidence of the
negative impact of adverse working conditions, insecure work, and unemployment on
mental and physical health. In contrast, it shows fair employment with decent working
conditions can enhance health and well-being. In addition, it provides evidence of the
need for social protection across the life course and in the case of specific shocks, such

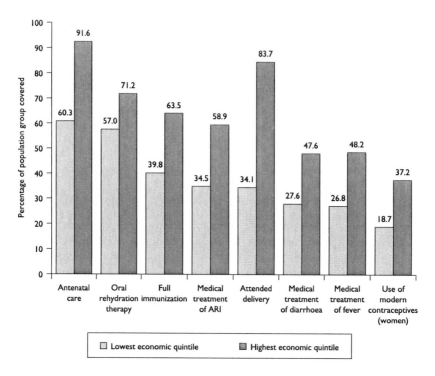

Figure 7.3 Use of basic maternal and child health services by lowest and highest economic quintiles, 50+ countries. Reproduced by permission of the World Bank

as illness, disability, and loss of income or work. Generous universal social protection systems are associated with better population health, including lower excess mortality among the old and lower mortality among socially disadvantaged groups.

Finally, this principle for action makes the case that the health care system is itself a social determinant of health, which is influenced by and influences the other social determinants. By way of illustration, Figure 7.3 shows the use of basic maternal and child health services by lowest and highest economic quintiles in 50+ countries. Consequently, the CSDH advocates universal health care coverage financed through general taxation and/or mandatory universal insurance. It stresses health care systems have better health outcomes when built on primary health care where prevention and promotion are in balance with investment in curative interventions (CSDH, 2008: 3–8).

Tackle the inequitable distribution of power, money, and resources

The second principle for action reflects the CSDH's conclusion that 'inequity in the conditions of daily living is shaped by deeper social structures and processes. The inequity is systematic, produced by social norms, policies, and practices that tolerate or actually promote unfair distribution of and access to power, wealth, and other necessary social resources' (CSDH, 2008: 10). The CSDH report cites evidence that government policies can either improve or worsen health and health equity and that in developing policies, governments need to adopt a 'health in all policies' approach that recognizes the breadth of the social determinants of health. In doing so, policy coherence between different government departments and policies is essential. Community engagement and social participation in the policy-making process are seen by the CSDH as crucial in that they help ensure decision-making is fair. The report also proposes that health can be used as a rallying point for different sectors and actors through the development of local health plans.

The CSDH also calls for public financing of action across the determinants of health as part of this second principle for action. It cites evidence that the socio-economic development of rich countries was strongly supported by publicly financed infrastructure and progressively universal public services. It also puts forward evidence that modest levels of income redistribution through progressive taxation have considerably greater impact on poverty reduction than economic growth alone. For poorer countries, it calls for much greater international financial assistance. The report also stresses that health is a matter of rights and a public sector responsibility. It cites evidence that the commercialization of vital social goods such as education, water, and health care leads to inequity. In addition, the CSDH underlines the importance of addressing gender inequities through its second principle for action.

> Gender inequities are pervasive in all societies. Gender biases in power, resources, entitlements, norms and values, and the way in which organizations are structured and programmes are run damage the health of millions of girls and women. The position of women in society is also associated with child health and survival – of boys and girls. Gender inequities influence health through, among other routes, discriminatory feeding patterns, violence against women, lack of decision-making power, and unfair divisions of work, leisure, and possibilities of improving one's life.
>
> (CSDH, 2008: 16)

Measure and understand the problem and assess the impact of action

The CSDH cites evidence that countries without basic data on mortality and morbidity by socio-economic indicators have difficulty addressing health inequities (Kelly and Mackenbach, 2007). Furthermore, those countries with the poorest data are those with the worst health problems. It also calls for action to build capacity on the social determinants among policy-makers, practitioners – including health and medical professionals – and other stakeholders.

The CSDH report concludes:

> This is a long-term agenda, requiring investment starting now, with major changes in social policies, economic arrangements, and political action. At the centre of this action should be the empowerment of people, communities, and countries that currently do not have their fair share. The knowledge and the means to change are at hand and are brought together in this report. What is needed now is the political will to implement these eminently difficult but feasible changes. Not to act will be seen, in decades to come, as failure on a grand scale to accept the responsibility that rests on all our shoulders.
>
> (CSDH, 2008: 23)

Addressing the social determinants of health through policy

One of the tasks of the CSDH was 'to foster a global movement' to promote health equity (CSDH, 2008: 3) and since its publication, the CSDH report has had considerable influence on policy at international and national level. At an international level, the member states of the WHO adopted a resolution at the World Health Assembly in May 2009 'Reducing health inequities through action on the social determinants of health'. The resolution called on member states, the WHO Secretariat, and the international community to implement the recommendations of the Commission, highlighting areas such as measurement of health inequities, implementing a social determinants of health approach in public health programmes, adopting a 'health in all policies approach' to government, and aligning work on the social determinants of health with the renewal of primary health care.

In October 2011, the World Conference on Social Determinants of Health was convened by the WHO and hosted by the Government of Brazil. The conference, which was attended by policy-makers and health leaders, focused on the importance and urgency of taking action on social determinants of health to reduce health inequities between and within countries. The conference adopted the Rio Political Declaration on Social Determinants of Health, which expresses global political commitment for the implementation of a social determinants of health approach to reduce health inequities and to achieve other global priorities. Priority areas include:

- Adopt better governance for health and development to tackle the root causes of, and to reduce, health inequities.
- Promote participation in policy-making and implementation for action on the social determinants of health, engaging actors and those with influence outside of government, including civil society.
- Further reorient the health sector towards reducing health inequities, including moving towards universal health coverage that is accessible, affordable, and good quality for all.
- Strengthen global governance and collaboration, including coordinated global action on the social determinants of health, aligned with national government policies and global priorities.
- Monitor progress and increase accountability to inform policies on the social determinants of health.

In May 2012, the Declaration was in turn adopted by WHO member states in a resolution which commits them to implement the pledges made in the priority areas.

There are also international initiatives at the regional level that reflect this increased emphasis on the need for action on the social determinants of health to reduce health inequities. For example, the WHO European Region has commissioned a major review of the social determinants of health and the health divide in the European Region, which covers 53 countries. The purpose of the review is to identify the relevance of the findings of the CSDH and other new evidence to the European context and translate these into policy proposals. The review will inform the new policy for health for the European Region, Health 2020 (WHO, 2011).

At a national level, governments have also adopted the social determinants of health approach to develop strategies to reduce inequalities in health. In England, for example, the government commissioned Michael Marmot, who chaired the CSDH, to chair an independent review to propose the most effective evidence-based strategies for reducing health inequalities in England from 2010. The final report, 'Fair Society Healthy Lives', was published in February 2010, and concluded that reducing health inequalities would require action on six policy objectives:

- Give every child the best start in life
- Enable all children, young people, and adults to maximize their capabilities and have control over their lives
- Create fair employment and good work for all
- Ensure a healthy standard of living for all
- Create and develop healthy and sustainable places and communities
- Strengthen the role and impact of ill-health prevention (Marmot, 2010).

Another example is the Spanish Government's adoption in 2008 of the theme to reduce health inequalities as a priority. To take this forward, a Commission on the Reduction of Social Inequalities in Health was established. It published a report proposing action on the social determinants of health in five domains:

1 Distribution of power, wealth and resources
2 Living and working conditions throughout the life cycle
3 Health-promoting environments
4 Health care
5 Information, monitoring, research and teaching (Government of Spain, 2010).

Implications for health promotion

Recognizing the social determinants of health as causes of health and well-being is crucial to effective health promotion. This chapter has shown that lifestyle and behaviour factors associated with health and ill health are strongly influenced by factors such as income, employment, education, environment, and social networks. Health promotion, therefore, needs to address these factors. This will mean more agencies, sectors, services, and individuals are implicated in health promotion because it requires action on all the social determinants of health. In addition, health must be included in all policies because all action has the potential to impact on health. This also requires ensuring congruence across the policy spectrum. Community participation in defining needs, designing solutions, and delivering these is crucial.

Understanding how unequal access to the social determinants of health contributes to health inequity is also important for designing interventions. For example, physical activity programmes and other health initiatives need to target communities that do not access existing services. If they do not, there is a danger health inequities will increase as the health of the population as a whole improves because they access these new services, while the physical and mental health of disadvantaged communities continues to lag further behind. However, focusing solely on the most disadvantaged will not reduce health inequalities sufficiently. To reduce the steepness of the social gradient in health, actions must be universal, but with a scale and intensity that is proportionate to the level of disadvantage. This approach is known as proportional universalism (CSDH, 2008; Marmot, 2010).

Finally, the social determinants approach has important implications for measuring the effectiveness of health promotion interventions. There may be significant time lags before action on these determinants results in improvements in health equity. This makes it more difficult to attribute causality and demonstrate effectiveness. This has led to calls for a rethinking of what constitutes 'evidence' and greater effort to improve, collect, and share this evidence (CSDH, 2008).

Activity 7.3

This activity encourages you to reflect on action on the social determinants of health in your country. Identify a policy or project that seeks to change the social determinants of health in your country. Describe how this will impact on health and suggest ways that these impacts could be measured. What issues are involved in assessing these impacts?

Feedback

You may have identified projects on the social determinants of health such as those related to employment, housing, income, education, gender equality, the environment, and access to services. You may have suggested impact be measured by process indicators (such as investment levels or having a strategy in place), service indicators (such as children going to school or people accessing training), and outcome measures (such as improvements in educational achievement or levels of unemployment). You may also have identified issues that complicate measuring the impact of specific interventions on health outcomes, including: the time lag between action and changes in health status; the difficulty in attributing change in health status to a single intervention; and the possibility of compounding factors.

Summary

This chapter has explored what determines health and models that have been proposed to explain how these determinants interact to influence health. It has also discussed the growing importance attached to the social determinants of health in policies to reduce inequities in health and the types of interventions these policies have proposed. Finally, the chapter has looked at the implications of this approach for health promotion practice.

References

Barker, D.J.P. (1998) *Mothers, Babies and Disease in Later Life* (2nd edn.). Edinburgh: Churchill Livingstone.

Bartley, M., Power, C., Blane, D., Davey Smith, G. and Shipley, M. (1994) Birth weight and later socioeconomic disadvantage: evidence from the 1958 British cohort study, *British Medical Journal*, 309: 1475–8.

Commission on Social Determinants of Health (CSDH) (2008) *Closing the Gap in a Generation: Health Equity through Action on the Social Determinants of Health*. Final Report of the Commission on Social Determinants of Health. Geneva: World Health Organization.

Dahlgren, G. and Whitehead, M. (1991) *Policies and strategies to promote social equity in health* (mimeo). Stockholm: Institute for Future Studies.

Government of Spain, Directorate General for Public Health and Foreign Health Ministry of Health (2010) *Moving Forward Equity: A Proposal of Policies and Interventions to Reduce Social Inequalities in Health in*

Spain. Madrid: Directorate General for Public Health and Foreign Health Ministry of Health. Available at: http://www.mspsi.gob.es/profesionales/saludPublica/prevPromocion/promocion/desigualdadSalud/docs/Moving_Forward_Equity.pdf [accessed 16 November 2012].

Graham, H. (2001) The Health Variations programme and the public health agenda, *Health Variations: The Official Newsletter of the ESRC Health Variations Programme*, Issue 7, April. Lancaster: Lancaster University.

Gwatkin, D.R., Wagstaff, A. and Yazbeck, A. (eds.) (2005) *Reaching the Poor with Health, Nutrition, and Population Services: What Works, What Doesn't, and Why.* Washington, DC: The World Bank.

Harris, E., Sainsbury, P. and Nutbeam, D. (eds.) (1999) *Perspectives on Health Inequity.* Sydney, NSW: Australian Centre for Health Promotion.

Kelly, M. and Mackenbach, J. (2007) *The Social Determinants of Health: Developing an Evidence Base for Political Action.* Final report to the World Health Organization, Commission on the Social Determinants of Health from Measurement and Evidence Knowledge Network. Chile: Universidad del Desarrollo/London: National Institute for Health and Clinical Excellence.

Lalonde, M. (1974) *A New Perspective on the Health of Canadians: A Working Document* (the Lalonde Report). Ottawa: Government of Canada.

Marmot, M. (2004) *Status Syndrome: How Our Position on the Social Gradient Affects Longevity and Health.* London: Bloomsbury.

Marmot, M. (2010) *Fair Society, Healthy Lives: Strategic Review of Health Inequalities in England Post 2010.* London: Marmot Review. Available at: www.marmotreview.org [accessed 16 November 2012].

Marmot, M.G., Rose, G., Shipley, M. and Hamilton, P.J.S. (1978) Employment grade and coronary heart disease in British civil servants, *Journal of Epidemiology and Community Health*, 32: 244–9.

McGinnis, J.M., Williams-Ruso, P. and Knickman, J.R. (2002) The case for more active policy attention to health promotion, *Health Affairs*, 21(2): 78–93.

Townsend, P., Davidson, N. and Whitehead, M. (1988) *Inequalities in Health: The Black Report and the Health Divide.* London: Pelican.

World Health Organization (WHO) (2011) *Interim Second Report on Social Determinants of Health and the Health Divide in the WHO European Region.* Copenhagen: WHO.

Further reading

Graham, H. (2004) Social determinants and their unequal distribution: clarifying policy understandings, *Millbank Quarterly*, 82(1): 101–24.

World Health Organization (WHO) (1998) *Health21: Health for All in the 21st Century.* Copenhagen: WHO Regional Office for Europe.

World Health Organization (WHO) (2003) *The Solid Facts: Social Determinants of Health.* Copenhagen: WHO.

8 Theorizing inequalities in health

Adam Fletcher

Overview

In this chapter, you will be introduced to the nature and extent of health inequalities, and will learn about a range of theoretical perspectives that have been put forward to explain these inequalities and inform health promotion approaches and methods.

Learning objectives

After reading this chapter, you will be able to:

- list different examples of social inequalities in health
- critically discuss theories that have been proposed to explain health inequalities
- identify potential responses to health inequalities

Key terms

Inequalities in health: Differences in health status between different populations and social groups.

Inequities in health: A term that can be used to describe inequalities in health that are deemed preventable.

Socio-economic status: An individual's place in the social hierarchy according to their level of income, education, occupation, and/or where they live.

Social epidemiology: The field of epidemiology that examines the social and spatial distribution of health outcomes and the social determinants of health outcomes.

What are inequalities in health?

The term 'health inequalities' refers to differences in health outcomes, including morbidity and mortality, across different population sub-groups and countries. The notion that belonging to a particular social group or living in a certain type of country predisposes individuals to unnecessarily poorer health and lower life expectancy is not a new one, and doubtless was apparent long before the accumulation of what would now be accepted as 'scientific evidence' (Scrambler, 2011). In the early 1840s, Friedrich Engels (1845) famously wrote about the unfair social patterning of disease in England according to social class and income level. Social epidemiologists now routinely quantify such inequalities in health outcomes. For example, the Department of Health (2010: 5) in England recently reported: 'People living in the poorest areas will, on average, die 7 years earlier than people living in richer areas and spend up to 17 more years living with poor health.'

Epidemiologists studying inequalities in health outcomes measure socio-economic status in a range of ways, for example based on individual and family income, educational qualifications, occupational status, housing tenure, and/or area-based deprivation. There is consistent evidence that those individuals with the lowest socio-economic classification have, on average, the worst health outcomes and die youngest irrespective of the measure of socio-economic status used (Link and Phelan, 1995). In her book on socio-economic inequalities in health, Hilary Graham concluded that, despite improvements in life expectancy overall, health improvements have been 'more rapid among those at the top than the bottom of the socioeconomic hierarchy' (Graham, 2007: 12). This pattern is also evident throughout high-income countries (Mackenbach, 2005). Sometimes the term 'health inequities' is used to describe inequalities in health that are preventable.

Significant health inequalities have also been observed between countries. In high-income countries such as Japan and Sweden, a girl born today has a life expectancy of over 80 years but life expectancy is still less than 50 years in several countries in sub-Saharan Africa (CSDH, 2008). Maternal mortality also varies dramatically between countries. For example, the risk of death for mothers is one in eight in Afghanistan compared with only 1 in 17,400 in Sweden (WHO, 2007). As in high-income countries, there are also stark differences in health outcomes within low-income countries, which are closely linked to poverty and social disadvantage. For example, maternal mortality is four times higher among the poor compared with the rich in Indonesia (Graham et al., 2004).

Inequalities do not simply exist between the very best-off and worst-off in a society, however; health inequalities have also been observed along a 'social gradient', whereby there is a linear increase in ill health and mortality with decreasing socio-economic position (Marmot, 2004). This gradient exists in all countries according to a variety of socio-economic status factors such as income, level of education, occupation status, and neighbourhood characteristics (CSDH, 2008). This means that the more favourable your circumstances are, the better your chances of enjoying good health and a longer life. An example of such a social gradient is shown in Figure 8.1, which shows the death rate (all causes) per 100,000 inhabitants in Scotland by gender and the deprivation category (DEPCAT) of the area people live in.

Research on health inequalities according to gender has also developed since the late 1960s (Annandale, 1998). Graham (2000) has suggested that 'being a woman' exacerbates the problems of social disadvantage, whereby low socio-economic status further 'expresses itself' in a gendered form with, for example, women from low socio-economic groups most likely to smoke. In addition to high rates of maternal mortality in low-income countries, women in low-income contexts are exposed to further health risks through gender violence. The following case study provides an example of gender inequalities.

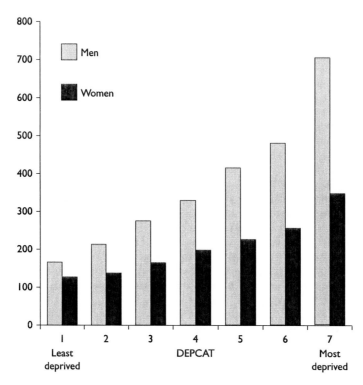

Figure 8.1 All-cause death rate per 100,000 population in Scotland. Reproduced under the terms of the Open Government Licence (OGL).

Box 8.1 Case study: Gender inequalities in HIV in sub-Saharan Africa

In sub-Saharan Africa, the rate of new HIV infections among women from the higher socio-economic groups has decreased since the start of the epidemic and HIV infections are now increasingly concentrated among the most disadvantaged and vulnerable young women (Hargreaves et al., 2008). This has been attributed to the investment in health education campaigns, which are most effective at reaching and changing the sexual-risk behaviour of women in higher socio-economic groups, while less educated women cannot always negotiate safer sexual practices owing to significant economic disadvantage, educational inequalities, and gender power imbalances within the region. Sexual violence is also common and is likely to be another important HIV risk factor in some conflict-affected settings. Analyses by researchers in the gender violence group at the London School of Hygiene & Tropical Medicine have found that such sexual violence could increase HIV incidence by 10 per cent (Watts et al., 2010).

Ethnicity is another axis of inequality that has received increasing attention, particularly in Europe (Bradby and Nazroo, 2010) and the USA (Bourgois, 1995). Inequalities in health outcomes, levels of health care service access, and in the quality of care experienced by minority ethnic groups all need to be urgently addressed throughout Europe and North America (WHO, 2010). As with gender, multiple dimensions of social and economic inequality overlap with ethnicity, and reinforce each other. For example, socio-economic disadvantage has been identified as a major reason why Afro-Caribbean communities have higher rates of poor health and chronic illness in the USA. The concentration of minority ethnic populations in specific geographical locations in countries such as the USA also has profound effects on their ability to access health services and benefit from public health improvement initiatives. However, not all social and cultural differences among minority ethnic groups have an adverse impact on health outcomes. For example, there is evidence that certain minority ethnic groups in the UK have a better mental health than the White British population, which may be attributable to family and community cultural factors among this group (see, for example, Goodman et al., 2008).

Activity 8.1

In this activity, you will reflect on health inequalities as they affect your own country.

1 What are the three main social axes through which health inequalities occur?
2 List examples of health inequalities from a country where you have lived.

Feedback

1 The three main social axes are: socio-economic status, gender, and ethnicity.

2 The Commission on the Social Determinants of Health (CSDH) was established by the World Health Organization (WHO) to address the social factors leading to ill health and inequalities in health globally. The final report published by the CSDH (2008) lists a wide range of examples of health inequalities between and within countries. These include obesity, malnutrition, mental health problems, heart disease, infant mortality, maternal death, diabetes, work-related health hazards, infectious diseases, injury and death from accidents, dental health, and the use of health-damaging commodities such as alcohol and tobacco. The report is recommended as further reading at the end of this chapter.

There has also been an increase in research examining not only how countries' health profiles vary according to their income levels but also how these appear to differ according to other societal level factors, particularly regarding how overall levels of income inequality may explain variations in different countries' health outcomes such as life expectancy. Wilkinson and Pickett (2009) analysed data from 21 high-income countries and found that irrespective of a nation's overall wealth, a narrower gap between rich and poor within a country is associated with better health and well-being in a population. They found that rich countries with the greatest levels of economic inequality such as the USA, the UK, and Portugal consistently have worse health outcomes and lower life expectancy than more equal countries such as Sweden, Norway, and Japan. The central implication is that more economic growth in a country will not lead to better health or well-being in these countries. In fact, there appears to be no discernible relationship between income per head and social well-being in high-income countries. However, making a country *more equal economically* can benefit the whole population in terms of reductions in violence, mental illness, obesity, drug use, teenage pregnancy, and other outcomes, as well as reduce health inequalities within a country. This research finding is illustrated in the case study below on international variations in child health and well-being.

Box 8.2   Case study: International variations in child health and well-being

In 2007, the United Nation's Children's Fund (UNICEF) drew on 40 indicators to systematically explore differences in child health and well-being reported across different high-income countries, including measures of family affluence, child health and safety, educational attainment, peer relationships, social and emotional well-being, and health-risk behaviours such as smoking, drinking, and drug use. The study concluded that children in countries such as the USA and the UK experienced the worst outcomes of all and those countries with the best child health and well-being outcomes were the most equal societies (see Figure 8.2).

The same was observed when looking at different aspects of child well-being and how this varies across different states of the USA (Wilkinson and Pickett, 2009). These studies both suggest that improvements in child well-being in rich societies will depend more on reductions in inequality than on further economic growth.

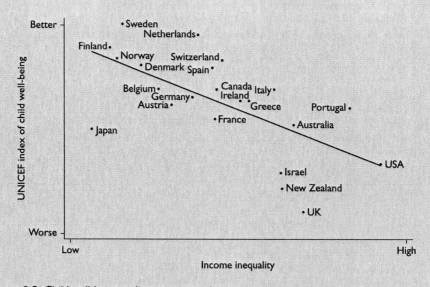

Figure 8.2 Child well-being and income inequality.

Source UNICEF (2007) *Child poverty in perspective: An overview of child well-being in rich countries.* Reproduced by permission of UNICEF

Policy responses to health inequalities

In the last decade, there has been some reconfiguring of the goals of public health policy, principally but not exclusively in developed countries, which has led to an increasing number of policy responses to health inequalities. Public health policies typically now emphasize the 'twin goals' of improving population health and reducing health inequalities. National and international policy documents, strategies, and frameworks that specifically focus on reducing differences in health outcomes between different social groups are now commonplace. For example, in the UK, *Saving Lives: Our Healthier Nation* was a government policy document launched with the specific aim of 'improving health for all and tackling health inequality' (Secretary of State for Health, 1999: 2). In the USA, a similar strategy launched a year later was 'designed to achieve two over-arching goals: increase quality and years of healthy life [and] *eliminate health disparities*' (USDHHS, 2000: 2). In North America, 'health disparities' is another term used to refer to the differences in health outcomes between different social groups and is therefore synonymous with 'health inequalities' in such contexts.

These British and American examples of public health policies are far from exceptional, and there are a growing number of examples of governments around the world developing comprehensive strategies to tackle inequalities. However, although increasingly commonplace, there is still little agreement in policy documents regarding the specific drivers of significant inequalities or clear priority areas for action. National policies instead tend to have a broad focus, often acknowledging all possible explanations with wide-ranging recommendations. To use the example of the UK again, in 2003, *Tackling Health Inequalities: A Programme for Action* (Department of Health, 2003) identified the need to address the wider social influences on health, including taking action in all the following areas: reducing levels of child poverty; improving the quality of poor housing; improving local transport; improving educational attainment and tackling low basic skills; tackling unemployment; and strengthening poor communities through improving access to social and community facilities and services.

At an international level, there has also been an increasing acknowledgement of what Link and Phelan (1995) termed the 'fundamental causes of disease' (also sometimes termed the 'causes of the causes' of disease), explicitly anchoring risky health behaviours in the context of a wide range of underlying social and material circumstances and structures. The World Health Organization has shown commitment to support action on inequalities, such as the Health21 strategy (WHO, 1999) with the aim of reducing the health gap between socio-economic groups within countries by at least a quarter in all member states to substantially improve the health of the most disadvantaged groups. Furthermore, the WHO Commission on the Social Determinants of Health committed later to the same aspiration globally. This is discussed in more detail in Chapter 7 on the determinants of health.

If the Health21 strategy was the beginning of the journey towards an international public policy agenda focused on health inequalities, then the recommendations of Michael Marmot and his team for the Commission on the Social Determinants of Health (CSDH, 2008) were intended to operationalize this at a global level. They concluded that reducing health inequalities would require action on six broad policy objectives to:

• give every child the best start in life
• enable all children, young people and adults to maximize their capabilities and have control over their lives
• create fair employment and good work for all

- ensure a healthy standard of living for all
- create and develop healthy and sustainable places and communities
- strengthen the role and impact of ill-health prevention.

What these wide-ranging national and international policy responses to health inequalities have in common is a lack of explicit use of *theory*. As Graham (2007: 13) observes of inequalities in health and policy responses to these, 'noting that the association persists is not, of course, the same thing as explaining how it persists'. Theories offer a framework for studying social problems and can provide explanations for the ways in which change occurs in individuals, communities, and societies. Health promoters therefore need theories to inform specific appropriate and effective interventions and programme planning. In other words, theories are fundamental to help answer such questions as: What inequalities exist between social groups? Who is affected? What are the causes of these inequalities? How should we address the causes? These questions remain a major blind-spot in policy documents to reduce health inequalities despite the wide range of theoretical explanations that have been advanced. The next section reviews these different explanations.

Activity 8.2

This activity encourages you to reflect on the types of policies governments have put in place to improve health and/or address health inequalities. Think about government health policies in your country. Do these policies explicitly address health inequalities or do they seek to improve health for the population as a whole? What is their focus and what are they seeking to change?

Feedback

Policies that seek to address health inequalities will target health changes among those individuals and communities that experience the poorest health outcomes, as opposed to general health policies, which are aimed at the population as a whole. For example, they could include policies that seek to: address unequal access to health services by improving services in isolated or deprived areas; reduce health-damaging behaviour such as smoking; or modify key social determinants of health (for example, low educational attainment).

Theories to explain health inequalities

This section describes seven different theoretical perspectives that have been used to try and explain the types of inequalities in health outcomes between social groups described in the first section of this chapter. Theories can help the design of more effective health promotion approaches and methods. However, as discussed above, there is often little agreement in policy circles regarding the relative merits and importance of these different theories. While the Black Report (Townsend and Davidson, 1980) in the UK was certainly an important catalyst for developing clearer theories regarding why the poorest people have such manifestly worse health outcomes, there are now multiple, sometimes competing, explanations. There is no comprehensive and non-contentious way of categorizing these explanations but seven different bodies of theories that have emerged are outlined in turn below.

Activity 8.3

This activity explores different theories that have been proposed to explain health inequalities. Seven different explanations put forward to better understand and theorize the drivers of health inequalities are described below. In order to revise the key points, for each explanation make a note of:

1 The influences on unequal health outcomes emphasized by that explanation.
2 The limitations and criticisms of each explanation. Also,
3 Consider what the main implications for intervention are for each of these different theoretical explanations.

Examples of the implications of each explanation are listed in the feedback section for this activity later in the chapter.

Material explanations

A central theoretical proposition has traditionally been that it is the material circumstances and conditions in which poorer people live that predisposes them to worse health and a shorter life expectancy. This material perspective therefore argues that it is these differences in people's material circumstances that explain the wide variations in health outcomes according to social axes such as socio-economic status. This has been based on the notion that a lack of income and economic disadvantage are thought to lead to a lack of food, inadequate housing, and poor sanitation, which, in turn, lead to worse health outcomes and a lower life expectancy among the lowest socio-economic groups. The employment conditions of the working poor may also put them at increased risk (for example, dangerous and dirty working environments). The strength of this theoretical perspective is that it focuses clearly on the importance of poverty, poor housing, and working conditions as major determinants of health. This is likely to be especially valid in low-income countries.

However, this theory, which was a strong theme in the seminal Black Report on health inequalities (Townsend and Davidson, 1980), is now thought to be too simplistic and unconvincing in most high-income countries, which have large welfare states and where relatively few people are living in 'absolute' poverty without access to food and shelter. Furthermore, material explanations are also limited in that they cannot adequately explain the social gradient consistently observed in key health outcomes. That is, it is not only the very poorest in material terms or those living and working in the very worst conditions who have the worst health outcomes, there is a linear increase in ill health and mortality with decreasing socio-economic status. For example, even excluding the poorest 5 per cent and the richest 5 per cent, the gap in life expectancy in England between low and high income is still 6 years, and in disability-free life expectancy 13 years (Department of Health, 2010). Material perspectives have also been criticized because they ignore other important determinants of early mortality and non-communicable disease in families and communities of lower socio-economic status, particularly smoking, alcohol consumption, and drug use.

Neo-materialist explanations

Neo-materialist explanations have emerged partly in response to the critiques and limitations of traditional material explanations. Rather than simply focusing on poverty and the living and working conditions of the poorest, the neo-material perspective emphasizes the importance of social policies and welfare provision more broadly, which can influence health outcomes. For example, the quality and accessibility of health services, state education, active transport initiatives, parks, and other community facilities are all likely to influence health outcomes. These neo-material explanations suggest that certain communities or regions have better social services and welfare provision and this explains the differences in life expectancy and other health outcomes between these areas. A key strength of this perspective is that it addresses some of the limitations of traditional, cruder material explanations, situating health inequalities in the context of public policies and recognizing the importance of 'place' (Popay and Williams, 2009). It also draws attention to what is known as the 'inverse care law', whereby the availability of good medical or social care has been found to vary inversely with the needs of the population served (Tudor Hart, 1971).

A major criticism with such perspectives is that in countries such as the UK, Canada, and Australia, health, education, and other social services are provided universally, thus potentially limiting the extent to which health inequalities can be attributed to differences in the receipt of these resources. Even if provision varies by area – a phenomenon that has been termed the 'post code lottery' (see, for example, Bungay, 2005) – this seems unlikely to fully explain either the social gradient observed in health outcomes or the extent of inequalities between the richest and poorest in many societies. It may be that neo-material explanations have greatest value in understanding inter-country differences in health outcomes whereby the most comprehensive welfare states, such as in Sweden, promote population-level health (Lynch et al., 2000). However, Wilkinson and Pickett (2009) largely argue against this and suggest that the differences observed in health outcomes between Western countries are more likely to be due to entrenched income and social inequalities (for example, in the USA and the UK) and *psycho-social factors* may have more explanatory value (described below). As with traditional material explanations, neo-material perspectives also largely ignore key determinants of early mortality in communities of low socio-economic status, such as smoking, and they do not specifically recognize the importance of certain stages of the life course (Bartley, 2003).

Cultural and behavioural explanations

Emanating from the Black Report (Townsend and Davidson, 1980), cultural and behavioural explanations have become a common starting point for theorists seeking to explain health inequalities. They emphasize how certain social classes and/or lower income groups often share a culture that promotes and reinforces certain 'risky' health-related behaviours (for example, smoking and poor diet) and inhibits other more health-promoting behaviours (for example, regular exercise and screening). A strength of these explanations is that in many high-income countries this resonates with the evidence regarding how groups of low socio-economic status have much higher rates of smoking, drinking, and poor dietary behaviours, and much lower life-expectancy. These explanations have also permeated popular discourses and 'lay' constructions of health inequalities (Popay et al., 2003).

Although a popular explanation, theories of health inequality that focus on cultural and behavioural phenomena have been criticized for ignoring poverty, income inequality, and other major 'upstream' structural determinants of health such as social exclusion and discrimination. Furthermore, social epidemiological studies have demonstrated that, while certain 'lifestyle risk factors' for early mortality are more prevalent in low-income communities, neither smoking nor other individual risks such as poor diet adequately explain socio-economic differences in mortality on their own (Shaw et al., 1999). In his review article for the journal *Sociology of Health and Illness*, Graham Scrambler (2011: 135) concluded that:

> In the 30 years since the publication of The Black Report it has become apparent that people's behaviours are often anchored not just in their culture but in their social and economic circumstances: eating healthily is not cheap and smoking can afford temporary relief in the face of the monotony of everyday lives devoid of tangible hope.

In short, these behavioural explanations tend to 'blame the victims' of wider structural inequalities, poverty, and social disadvantage. There is also increasing evidence regarding the importance of these more 'upstream' influences on health. For example, interventions that only aim to address these behavioural determinants by improving knowledge, skills, and modifying norms are often found to have only limited effects (Marmot, 2010; Chokshi and Farley, 2012), particularly for those at greatest risk (White et al., 2009). While this highlights the need to address material factors and neo-materialist redistribution, there is also now increasing interest in the 'psychosocial' and how individuals' experiences of relative poverty and social position determine unequal health outcomes within and across affluent societies.

Psychosocial explanations

Psychosocial 'risk factors' have also been used to develop theories to explain inequalities in health according to socio-economic status and income. Advocates of such psychosocial explanations tend to focus on 'the ramifications of social inequality' for how people see, define, and evaluate themselves and their behaviours. For example, Michael Marmot (2004) has drawn on evidence from the British 'Whitehall studies', in which researchers followed cohorts of civil servants over 30 years, to argue that people's sense of control and subjective sense of their social positioning is what is salient for their health and this explains the marked differences in health outcomes observed between different social and economic groups. Richard Wilkinson's seminal studies of health inequalities across different countries have complemented Marmot's theoretical position – first, by suggesting that income inequality leads to social fragmentation, and a breakdown in social support and trust, which damage health and well-being (Wilkinson, 1996); and second, by developing the notion of 'social comparison' and its importance for understanding how a subjective sense of positioning within the social hierarchy is a critical determinant of long-term health outcomes (Wilkinson and Pickett, 2009).

A major strength of this theoretical approach is the explicit recognition that material/'neo-material' circumstances and cultural traits cannot on their own fully explain the gradient in health observed by social position, which is currently observed in many high-income countries. There is also support for the importance of individuals' hierarchical position in the work environment and in society more generally from empirical studies (Marmot, 2004; Wilkinson and Pickett, 2009). However, while these psychosocial explanations do not ignore the environment around individuals, they potentially underestimate the importance and multiplicity of the wider social and material determinants of health. For example, childhood obesity may be concentrated among the poorest families because 'fast food' is cheap and easy to access in these areas, because there are fewer safe places to engage in physical activity in the neighbourhood where these families live, or because these behaviours are socially learned and promoted within the local culture, school or family environment. In other words, focusing on social hierarchies largely ignores these other equally important dimensions, limiting its explanatory value for many health behaviours. It is also unclear exactly why some people are more 'susceptible' than others to poor health due to their social status, or how factors such as lower employment status and limited social support are influential and effects occur, although it has been suggested the having less status and autonomy leads to greater stress and, in turn, worse health outcomes (Marmot, 2004).

Radical political theories

Radical theories of the 'political economy of health' and neo-Marxist 'theories of the state', which are based on the premise that certain social groups are actively discriminated against and marginalized, have also been drawn on to explain why health inequalities are reproduced. The political economy of health is a radical perspective that has emerged specifically to understand the conditions that shape population health and health service development within the wider macro-economic and political context (Doyle and Pennell, 1979). This perspective suggests that people's health is exchanged for economic growth (such as mining 'accidents' and unhealthy urban 'slum' environments) and the unequal disease burden is the 'price' of economic growth. This raises further questions regarding the balance between promoting economic growth and health, and draws attention to whose health is 'consumed' and 'transformed into wealth' and for whom (Doyle and Pennell, 1979). Public health researchers such as Phillipe Bourgois (1995) have also drawn on radical Marxist traditions in social research to emphasize how poverty, social exclusion, and racial discrimination can shape health outcomes such as drug-related harm and violence.

Although they draw important attention to the role of political actors in shaping health inequalities in addition to the role of behaviours of individuals' 'lifestyles' in low-income communities, macro-level political explanations are not strong biologically, particularly as all disease does not automatically correlate with socio-economic status or simply follow a pattern whereby poverty equates to increased risk (for example, HIV in sub-Saharan Africa was more common among more educated, higher income groups early in the epidemic). This evidence therefore counters arguments for a grand overall vulnerability approach. Nonetheless, political actors will shape material and social conditions, which in turn influence health, but different political ideologies, actions, and social conditions are likely to vary over space and time and in different epidemiological contexts. This inhibits the explanatory value of such theories, which are overly deterministic and ignore the role of individual agency, different policy environments, and complex casual pathways.

Natural selection

Some have argued that inequalities in health are due to a process whereby the least healthy people end up with the lowest incomes and in the lowest social classes – a process known as 'selection', which was discussed in the Black Report (Townsend and Davidson, 1980). This may be via *direct selection*, whereby those people who are unhealthy end up in the lowest social classes/income groups specifically because of their health status. It may also be due *indirectly* to personality and behavioural traits that are associated with poor health and mean that the least healthy people end up in the lowest social classes/income groups – that is, not directly because of their health status, but indirectly through these personal traits or behavioural confounders. In this theory, socio-economic status is therefore considered the dependent (rather than the independent) variable and health is given more causal significance. Thus, it is argued that a class system acts essentially as a 'filter' for people and sorts them according to many assets, one of which is health. In this scenario, the healthiest people are largely in the most affluent class, whereas those who have, or are more prone to, worse health outcomes, 'sink' towards lower groups of lower socio-economic status.

The notion of 'selection' has the advantage of taking a life-course perspective and it emphasizes the importance of early health and development for long-term social, economic, and health outcomes in later life. However, the theory of 'selection' cannot be regarded as a major explanation for social inequalities in health (Manor et al., 2003). In particular, it is highly implausible for explaining most of the health inequalities that have emerged and persist globally because there is simply rarely enough social mobility – that is, movement of people between groups of different socio-economic status – to explain differences in health status between different populations and social groups. If anything, the opposite is true, with social and economic hierarchies becoming more entrenched over time so the current generation of young people often have less social mobility than ever before (OECD, 2008).

Artefact explanations

Some have suggested that both health and socio-economic status are artificial variables, which have arisen as part of an attempt to measure social phenomena, and that the relationship between them may be an artefact and have no causal significance. Such explanations tend to point out that over time there are fewer people in the poorest social classes and therefore this accounts for the persistence of health inequalities. The theory argues that because of poor data, it is hard to determine whether there is a relationship between social class and health over time. However, research has consistently shown that other indicators of disadvantage, such as housing tenure, level of education, and income, all show a similar pattern of health inequalities, which would suggest that inequalities in health are not an artefact (Link and Phelan, 1995). Nonetheless, measuring social class accurately is important both in terms of being able to monitor the existence of health inequalities and to find ways of reducing them. While improving such measures is important, very few people accept inadequacies or errors in the measurement of social class can explain all the inequalities observed.

Activity 8.3 Feedback

There will never be one answer to tackling health inequalities. Successful strategies will assess fully the range and nature of inequalities that exist and apply a range of solutions to fit the context. Health promotion strategies therefore need to be multi-faceted, long term, and address key phases in the life course. These different theoretical explanations all highlight different areas for potential intervention:

Material explanations
The main implication is that there should be greater emphasis on addressing poverty and other aspects of material deprivation through social policies, such as redistributive cash transfers to those living in relative poverty and the provision of high-quality social housing for those that cannot afford it through the private market.

Neo-material explanations
A central implication is that social policies that promote high-quality, universal welfare provision can reduce health inequalities, such as the 'Scandinavian model'. These explanations also suggest the importance of Health Impact Assessments (HIA) at a community or regional level to assess the impact of public policies on health.

Cultural and behavioural explanations
Various health promotion approaches and methods may be appropriate to address these cultural and behavioural drivers of poor health in families, schools, and communities of lower socio-economic status, such as community mobilization interventions that aim to change social norms and targeted health education or mass media campaigns.

Psychosocial explanations
Interventions and policies that aim to promote individuals social capital and social support are implied here. A broader implication is to reduce social inequality, as one of the consequences is an increase in these psychosocial 'risk factors'. At a more proximal level, interventions aiming to empower individuals and reduce stress in the workplace may be appropriate.

Radical political theories
The central implication of these theories is for more radical approaches and this would potentially involve changing political and economic structures. In the extreme this could involve the overthrow of capitalism, but more feasibly it might involve reforms to voting systems, more direct democracy, and 'structural' interventions that address deep-rooted material disadvantages such as much greater cash transfers to those living in poverty.

Natural selection
Interventions to promote children's and young people's health and reduce absence from school at a young age may be relevant, as might anti-discrimination legislation to ensure those people with chronic health conditions and disability can find employment and be supported in work and the community. However, these measures on their own will likely have little effect on social mobility.

Artefact explanations
There are no practical implications for intervention as these explanations are based on the premise that there is no real relationship between socio-economic status and health outcomes, although few people accept this.

Summary

Health inequalities persist globally, both between and within countries. Socio-economic status, gender, and ethnicity are the major axes of inequality in health within countries. These are not biologically determined or a matter of chance but are shaped in complex ways by the actions of individuals and their families and friends, schools-and communities, and governments and other policy-makers. A wide range of explanations has emerged and are summarized in this chapter. Several of these explanations are particularly important for understanding how health inequalities occur and persist, such as those focused on material and neo-material circumstances, cultural and behavioural factors, and psychosocial concepts, and these should be the focus of coordinated health promotion interventions at key stages in the life course. Action to reduce health inequalities thus means taking a holistic approach, going beyond the health sector, and tackling these factors through public policy using a range of health promotion methods and approaches. Such action also needs to be more fully theorized regarding how it will reduce health inequalities.

References

Annandale, E. (1998) Health, illness and the politics of gender, in D. Field and S. Taylor (eds.) *Sociological Perspectives on Health, Illness and Health Care*. Oxford: Blackwell Science.

Bartley, M. (2003) *Health Inequality: An Introduction to Theories, Concepts and Methods*. Cambridge: Polity Press.

Bourgois, P. (1995) *In Search of Respect: Selling Crack in El Barrio*. New York: Cambridge University Press.

Bradby, H. and Nazroo, J. (2010) Health, ethnicity and race, in W. Cockerham (ed.) *The New Blackwell Companion to Medical Sociology*. Oxford: Wiley-Blackwell.

Bungay, H. (2005) Cancer and health policy: the postcode lottery of care, *Social Policy and Administration*, 39: 35–48.

Chokshi, D.A. and Farley, T.A. (2012) The cost-effectiveness of environmental approaches to disease prevention, *New England Journal of Medicine*, 367: 295–7.

Commission on Social Determinants of Health (CSDH) (2008) *Closing the Gap in a Generation: Health Equity through Action on the Social Determinants of Health*. Final Report of the Commission on Social Determinants of Health. Geneva: World Health Organization.

Department of Health (DoH) (2003) *Tackling Health Inequalities: A Programme for Action*. London: The Stationery Office.

Department of Health (DoH) (2010) *Healthy Lives, Healthy People: Our Strategy for Public Health in England*. London: The Stationery Office.

Doyle, L. and Pennell, I. (1979) *The Political Economy of Health*. London: Pluto Press.

Engels, F. (1845/1987) *The Condition of the Working Class in England*. Harmondsworth: Penguin.

Goodman, A., Patel, V. and Leon, D. (2008) Child mental health differences amongst ethnic groups in Britain: a systematic review, *BMC Public Health*, 8: 258.

Graham, H. (2000) Socio-economic change and inequalities in men and women's health in the UK, in E. Annandale and K. Hunt (eds.) *Gender Inequalities in Health*. Buckingham: Open University.

Graham, H. (2007) *Unequal Lives: Health and Socioeconomic Inequalities*. Maidenhead: Open University Press.

Graham, W.J., Fitzmaurice, A.E., Bell, J.S. and Cairns, J.A. (2004) The familial technique for linking maternal death with poverty, *Lancet*, 363: 23–7.

Hargreaves, J., Bonell, C., Boler, T., Boccia, D., Birdthistle, I., Fletcher, A. et al. (2008) Systematic review exploring time-trends in the association between educational attainment and risk of HIV infection in sub-Saharan Africa, *AIDS*, 22: 403–14.

Link, B. and Phelan, J. (1995) Social conditions as fundamental causes of disease, *Journal of Health and Social Behaviour*, 35: 80–94.

Lynch, J.W., Smith, G.D., Kaplan, G.A. and House, J.S. (2000) Income inequality and mortality: importance to health of individual income, psychosocial environment, or material conditions, *British Medical Journal*, 320: 1200–4.

Mackenbach, J. (2005) *Health Inequalities: Europe in Profile*. Rotterdam: Erasmus MC University Medical Centre.

Manor, O., Matthews, S. and Power, C. (2003) Health selection: the role of inter- and intra-generational mobility on social inequalities in health, *Social Science and Medicine*, 57: 2217–27.

Marmot, M. (2004) *Status Syndrome: How Our Position on the Social Gradient Affects Longevity and Health*. London: Bloomsbury.

Marmot, M. (2010) *Fair Society, Healthy Lives: Strategic Review of Health Inequalities in England Post 2010*. London: Marmot Review. Available at: www.marmotreview.org [accessed 16 November 2012].

Organization for Economic Cooperation and Development (OECD) (2008) *Growing Unequal? Income Distribution and Poverty in OECD Countries*. Paris: OECD.

Popay, J. and Williams, G. (2009) Equalizing the people's health: a sociological perspective, in J. Gabe and M. Calnan (eds.) *The New Sociology of the Health Service*. London: Routledge.

Popay, J., Bennett, S., Thomas, C., Williams, G., Gatrell, A. and Bostock, L. (2003) Beyond 'beer, fags, egg and chips'? Exploring lay understandings of social inequalities in health, *Sociology of Health and Illness*, 25: 1–23.

Scottish Government (2008) *Equally Well: Report of the Ministerial Task Force on Health Inequalities*. Edinburgh: Scottish Government.

Scrambler, G. (2011) Health inequalities, *Sociology of Health and Illness*, 34: 130–46.

Secretary of State for Health (1999) *Saving Lives: Our Healthier Nation*. London: The Stationery Office.

Shaw, M., Dorling, D., Gordon, D. and Davey-Smith, G. (1999) *The Widening Gap: Health Inequalities and Policies in Britain*. Bristol: Policy Press.

Townsend, P. and Davidson, N. (eds.) (1980) *Inequalities in Health: The Black Report*. Harmondsworth: Penguin.

Tudor Hart, J. (1971) The inverse care law, *Lancet*, 297: 405–12.

United Nations Children's Fund (UNICEF) (2007) *Child Poverty in Perspective: An Overview of Child Well-being in Rich Countries*. Innocenti Report Card 7. Florence: UNICEF.

US Department of Health and Human Services (USDHHS) (2000) *Healthy People 2000*. Washington, DC: USDHHS.

Watts, C.H., Foss, A.M., Hossain, M., Zimmerman, C., von Simson, R. and Klot, J. (2010) Sexual violence and conflict in Africa: prevalence and potential impact on HIV incidence, *Sexually Transmitted Infections*, 86: 93–9.

White, M., Adams, J. and Heywood, P. (2009) How and why do interventions that increase health overall widen inequalities within populations?, in S.J. Babones (ed.) *Social Inequality and Public Health*. Bristol: Policy Press.

Wilkinson, R. (1996) *Unhealthy Societies: The Afflictions of Inequality*. London: Routledge.

Wilkinson, R. and Pickett, K. (2009) *The Spirit Level: Why More Equal Societies Almost Always Do Better*. London: Penguin.

World Health Organization (WHO) (1999) *Health21: The Health for All Policy Framework for the WHO European Region*. Copenhagen: WHO Regional Office for Europe.

World Health Organization (WHO) (2007) *Maternal Mortality in 2005: Estimates Developed by WHO, UNICEF, UNFPA and the World Bank*. Geneva: WHO.

World Health Organization (WHO) (2010) *How Health Systems Can Address Health Inequities Linked to Migration and Ethnicity*. Copenhagen: WHO Regional Office for Europe.

Further reading

Commission on Social Determinants of Health (CSDH) (2008) *Closing the Gap in a Generation: Health Equity through Action on the Social Determinants of Health*. Final Report of the Commission on Social Determinants of Health. Geneva: World Health Organization.

Wilkinson, R. and Marmot, M. (2003) *Social Determinants of Health: The Solid Facts*. Copenhagen: WHO.

Wilkinson, R. and Pickett, K. (2007) The problems of relative deprivation: why some societies do better than others, *Social Science and Medicine*, 65(9): 1965–78.

The Rose hypothesis: advantages of whole population over targeted approaches

9

Adam Fletcher, Liza Cragg and Anis Kazi

Overview

This chapter introduces the Rose hypothesis and describes both whole population and targeted approaches. Geoffrey Rose argued the risk of disease in a population is usually 'normally' distributed (Rose, 1981). If this is the case, more cases of a disease will arise among the large number of people at low or medium risk than the relatively small number of people deemed at 'high risk', which in turn has implications for how we design interventions to improve health at a population level. In particular, Rose highlights the limitation of only targeting high-risk groups and suggests that health promotion should focus more on shifting the level of risk for the whole population. This is known as the 'Rose hypothesis'. This chapter also considers some of the other benefits, as well as drawbacks, of both these approaches, including the 'prevention paradox', which is associated with population-level approaches.

Learning objectives

After reading this chapter, you will be able to:

- describe the Rose hypothesis and its implications for health promotion
- consider the implications of shifting the distribution of risk for whole populations, and give examples of public health policies and interventions that adopt this approach
- understand the difference between whole population and targeted interventions
- critically discuss the practical, ethical, and political challenges to whole population strategies which aim to reduce exposure to risk

Key terms

Iatrogenic effect: An unintentional harmful effect of an intervention or policy.

Prevention paradox: The paradoxical situation whereby a preventative measure that significantly benefits the whole population offers little to each individual.

Rose hypothesis: Proposition by Geoffrey Rose that, because risk is normally distributed on a continuum, prevention strategies focusing on the whole population are likely to be more effective than those focused on high-risk groups and individuals.

Targeted approach: A health promotion strategy or intervention targeted at individuals or groups who are identified as being at higher than average risk of disease, injury or other adverse health outcomes.

Whole population approach: A health promotion strategy or intervention aimed at the whole population in question, rather than targeted at specific high-risk individuals or groups. Also sometimes known as a 'universal' or 'population-level' approach.

The distribution of risk

Understanding how the risk of disease is distributed in the population is essential for designing effective health promotion strategies. Geoffrey Rose (1981) examined major public health problems, such as cardiovascular disease, and found that risk is usually normally distributed. This means that the distribution of risk for disease and mortality tends to follow a continuum in which the small proportion of people at high risk are at the extreme end. Consequently, the vast majority of the population who are considered to be at low to medium risk contribute to more 'cases' of disease overall than the relatively small number who are at high risk. Figure 9.1 illustrates this normal risk distribution.

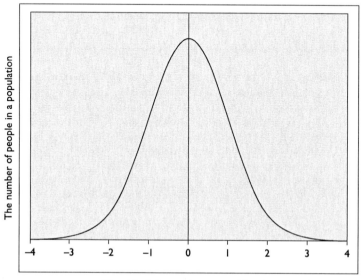

The risk of disease shown as a risk ratio

Figure 9.1 The normal distribution of risk. Reproduced with permission of Txt4Baby.

As a result of this 'normal' risk distribution, Geoffrey Rose (1985) proposed that strategies which seek to reduce risk as a whole within 'sick populations', rather than targeting a small proportion of high-risk individuals, will be more effective at improving health at a population level. The aim of such a whole population approach, also known in social policy as a universal approach, is therefore to shift the whole distribution of risk at a population level, rather than bringing those above a certain, usually arbitrary, risk threshold below it.

Targeted approaches, their limitations for improving health at a population level, and other problems associated with targeting, including the practical challenges of identifying high-risk groups and the potential for stigmatization, are discussed below. This is followed by a more detailed explanation of the advantages of whole population approaches over targeting, drawing on the examples used by Geoffrey Rose and others to illustrate this. Finally, the 'prevention paradox' and other limitations with the 'population approach' are outlined to critically discuss the strengths and limitations of the health promotion strategy advocated by Rose.

The targeted approach and its limitations

A targeted approach assumes that because some individuals and groups are at greater risk of health harms through disease or injury, they need specially targeted interventions. These individuals and groups may be considered more at risk because of age, gender, socio-economic status, disability, sexuality, genetic factors, or various lifestyle factors including diet, smoking, level of alcohol intake, and exercise.

The advantage of targeting certain individuals and groups considered to be at high risk is that the intervention is highly appropriate at that time for the individual concerned. This means that the individual may be more likely to be motivated to participate in a proposed intervention. For example, an individual diagnosed as being obese and having high cholesterol, and as a consequence at increased risk of coronary heart disease, may be more likely to respond to a behaviour change intervention relating to diet and exercise than someone who does not have similar risk factors and is at relatively low risk. A targeted approach also allows health care professionals to feel confident that the patient concerned has been given advice tailored to their diagnosis. The approach therefore seems to offer the opportunity for effective use of limited resources, as it focuses these resources on patients identified as being at high risk.

However, based on his analysis of the distribution of cardiovascular risk and the determinants of other major public health problems, Rose concluded:

> The preventive strategy that concentrates on high-risk individuals may be appropriate for those individuals, as well as being a wise and efficient use of limited medical resources; but its ability to reduce the burden of disease in the whole community tends to be disappointingly small. Potentially far more effective, and ultimately the only acceptable answer, is the mass strategy, whose aim is to shift the whole population's distribution of the risk variable.
>
> (Rose, 1981: 1851)

Without such a 'mass strategy', health promoters miss the majority of the population who will go on to experience the adverse health outcome that they are trying to prevent. In addition, there are several further disadvantages of approaches that only target high-risk individuals or groups, which have been discussed by Geoffrey Rose (1985) and others (e.g. Bonell and Fletcher, 2008) and are summarized below.

First, it is often difficult to define the boundaries of a 'high-risk' group and practically identify such individuals. Moreover, an individual's behaviour, lifestyle, and membership of social groups is dynamic, and these may change over the life course, which means 'risk' cannot easily be categorized or accurately monitored as people move from being high to medium or low risk. In addition, it is challenging to ensure that health promotion interventions and services engage high-risk individuals and groups, as these are often the hardest people to reach. At the same time, it is also not always possible to exclude others who are not specifically defined as 'at risk' from using these services. Furthermore, identifying some individuals and groups as high risk on an *ad hoc* basis via high-profile public health campaigns may result in those not identified believing they face no risk at all, leading them to ignore general health promotion advice.

Second, focusing only on those defined as at high risk also tends to ignore the social, economic, and environmental factors, often termed 'social determinants', which influence health and health inequalities. These social determinants of health are discussed in Chapter 7 of this book. Targeting high-risk individuals largely ignores the extent to which individuals' attitudes and behaviours are also influenced by wider societal, community, and peer group norms. Consequently, interventions targeted at small, high-risk groups have been criticized as 'palliative' and 'temporary' (Rose, 1985).

Finally, interventions that specifically target individuals deemed to be at high risk can have negative, harmful effects because they stigmatize such groups through 'labelling' them and/or aggregating together 'risky' groups and individuals (Bonell and Fletcher, 2008). Such unintentional harmful effects are known as iatrogenic effects in the fields of medicine and public health.

Activity 9.1

In this activity, you will consider interventions that are targeted at high-risk individuals. Think of an example of a strategy or intervention in your own country that seeks to address a problem by targeting individuals or groups at high risk? What is the intervention trying to achieve? Who is it targeting and how does it seek to reach this group? What might the difficulties be? Why is a targeted approach used for this problem?

Feedback

You might have considered interventions and strategies that include:

- Interventions to reduce teenage pregnancies and/or sexually transmitted infections among young women deemed to be at 'high risk'. They may be targeted through outreach youth work or through schools. Problems may include identifying who is at risk and the stigmatizing effects of participation.
- Interventions to reduce alcohol intake among problem drinkers. They could be targeted through GP and hospital services or through the criminal justice system. Problems include how to identify who is a problem drinker and reaching those that do not present to other services. The vast majority of alcohol-related harm at a population level would also be missed by such approaches.

- Interventions to encourage obese people to lose weight. These people could be targeted through GP and hospital services. As above, problems include reaching those that do not present to other services and ignoring wider societal level problems and norms regarding body weight.
- Interventions to reduce drug-related harm among young people. High-risk individuals could be targeted through health services, including drug treatment and harm reduction facilities, or through courts. However, this would most likely have little effect on population-level drug-related harm and could further stigmatize those groups targeted.

A targeted approach is generally used because it is considered that small groups are at much higher risk than the population as a whole of experiencing a particular health problem. It may be a low-cost option for intervention compared with population-level approaches and can allow politicians and other policy-makers to be seen to be doing something in the face of public concerns (Fletcher et al., 2012).

The whole population or universal approach

Owing to the limitations of targeting individuals and groups at high risk for promoting the health of a 'sick population', Geoffrey Rose instead proposed that prevention activities target a whole population regardless of variation in individuals' risk status. He argued that preventing disease by trying to shift the population-level distribution of a risk factor is more efficient than focusing interventions solely on people at high risk (Rose, 1985). For example, the Framingham Study found that lowering blood pressure by 10 per cent in the whole population caused a 30 per cent reduction in total attributable mortality (Stokes et al., 1989). To take diabetes as another example, there is no threshold between normal and hyper-glycaemic states but rather an increasing risk of neuropathy or retinopathy (nervous system damage or impaired vision) where there are uncontrolled levels of glucose in the body for a long period of time. The benefits of treating this with drugs will depend on the balance of side-effects against therapeutic benefits. Thus, in principle, decreasing glucose levels across a population would result in a larger decrease in the number of cases and the resultant disease prevalence than focusing attention on a small number of people with very high levels of blood glucose. Other examples of addressing the whole population are generic mass screening and vaccination programmes.

The whole population approach is centred on achieving change in the underlying causes that make the disease in question common in that population. This can be done through action on two broad levels. First, action on the social determinants of health, including focusing on more 'upstream' risk factors, for example through the provision of new public services, legislation to ban smoking, and healthy transport policies. And second, actions to change individuals' knowledge, attitudes, and behaviours, also sometimes termed more 'downstream' (or 'proximal') risk factors, for example through mass public health education.

The prevention paradox

Geoffrey Rose (1985) himself identified that a major challenge to universal approaches, which assume that the whole population is 'unhealthy', is that preventative interventions that benefit the whole population significantly may still only have a very small effect on most individuals or their risk of disease. This is what he terms the 'prevention paradox'. Consequently, those individuals may not consider some universal interventions worthwhile. Individuals are generally more motivated by their personal perceptions of benefit or risk rather than that of the wider population and are, therefore, less likely to participate in interventions they perceive as having little personal relevance for themselves. This can lead to the low take-up of and inconsistent adherence to whole population interventions. Examples include some health screening and vaccination programmes and the use of helmets for cycling. As Rose himself put it:

> The population strategy of prevention has also some weighty drawbacks. It only offers a small benefit to each individual, since most of them were going to be all right anyway, at least for many years. This leads to the Prevention Paradox: 'A preventive measure which brings much benefit to the population offers little to each participating individual'. This has been the history of public health – of immunization, the wearing of seat belts and now the attempt to change various life-style characteristics. Of enormous potential importance to the population as a whole, these measures offer very little – particularly in the short term to each individual; and thus there is poor motivation of the subject.
>
> (Rose, 1985: 38)

This lack of motivation is sometimes reinforced by public cynicism and lay epidemiology. For example, individual people and different communities may have their own perceptions of the effects of smoking, drinking alcohol, and eating high-fat foods that further entrenches their disengagement with whole population strategies (Popay et al., 2003). Some commentators have also suggested that the prevention paradox is exacerbated by the simplified messages about risk and adverse affects that many population-level health initiatives use. The failure to acknowledge the prevention paradox more directly in health education and promotion material can lead, at best, to greater mistrust among the general public of the messages contained, and at worst to their outright rejection (Davison et al., 1991).

Other limitations of whole population approaches

The Rose hypothesis is based on the underlying assumption that risk is normally distributed. It does not hold where risk is not normally distributed. One example of where risk is often not normally distributed is HIV/AIDS risk-behaviours, which tend to be concentrated among high-risk groups in many high-income countries, such as men who have sex with men and people who inject drugs. Where risk is not normally distributed but highly concentrated among certain vulnerable groups, targeted interventions are required.

There are also some situations where the whole population approach to prevention puts the health of some individuals at risk because a type of behaviour change that is appropriate for most of the population is not appropriate for the minority (Adams and White, 2005). For example, it has been suggested that a small amount of alcohol (red wine) has protective benefits. Consequently, a population-level reduction in the number of alcohol units drunk might increase risk for those people who have more benefit than risk from low-level consumption. Another example relates to body weight; population-level reductions in body weight will most likely be harmful for those people in a population who already have a very low body mass index. In these scenarios, the population distribution of risk shows what is called a 'J-shaped curve' (Adams and White, 2005).

There are also instances where a population approach may expose many people to a small risk. In these instances, the harm it could do may potentially outweigh the benefits, if these benefits are relatively minor. The 'MMR scare' in 1998 in the UK, where an association was deemed to have been found between the vaccination offered to all infants as protection against mumps, measles, and rubella and brain damage, is an example of when the perceived 'benefit to risk ratio' became increasingly worrisome for individuals and limited the scope for a population-level approach until the association was shown to be false (McIntyre and Leask, 2008).

The whole population approach has also been criticized for potentially exacerbating health inequalities because it does not address the underlying mechanisms that lead to different distributions of risk in different social groups and the fact that risk factors are concentrated among vulnerable and disadvantaged populations throughout the life course. This means that vulnerable groups are the 'least able to positively respond to population approach interventions' (Frohlich and Potvin, 2008: 219). Furthermore, if vulnerable groups who experience higher levels of risk do not participate in interventions that shift the distribution of a risk factor in a population as a whole, these interventions may maintain the inequalities that are present in the society, or even widen the gap. An example is educational interventions and other campaigns against smoking in the workplace (Lorenc et al., 2013). However, it is possible to shift the risk distribution at a population level and simultaneously reduce the differential between the richest and poorest in a society (Lorenc et al., 2013).

The population approach has also been challenged as lacking a clear theoretical base and supporting evidence. It has been suggested that it arises from an interpretive error known as the 'ecological fallacy', whereby inferences are made about individuals based on aggregate data for a group. As Charlton (1995: 609) put it, 'the population approach attempts to dispense with scientific understanding of causal processes, and base prevention upon a "theory-free" (black box) process of observation and manipulations'.

Implications for health promotion

The limitations of targeting individuals and groups deemed to be at high risk, which are described above, can be seen as a strong argument for a whole population approach to health promotion, also known as a universal approach. This approach aims to lower the levels of risk in the population as a whole to reduce the incidence of disease and improve health. This supports the use of complex social interventions and public policies that address the social determinants that influence the distribution of risk in a population. Such policies can include neighbourhood regeneration, active transport policies, measures to increase income redistribution, and the provision and expansion of universal education and other public services (Fletcher, 2013).

In addition to addressing these upstream factors, whole population, universal approaches can also address individuals' knowledge, attitudes, and health-related behaviours via mass interventions that are aimed at everybody in a country or region. These individual-level factors, such as knowledge and attitudes, are termed downstream risk factors. Interventions to address them include mass health education programmes and media campaigns. In addition, the World Health Organization advocates for global adolescent health improvement through greater intervention in schools. This is not only because schools are well-resourced settings and children and young people attend school during a critical period when key health risk behaviours increase markedly (Viner et al., 2012), but also because schools provide access to the vast majority of children and young people. Consequently, effective school-based health improvement interventions have the potential to produce significant population-level health improvements.

Activity 9.2

In this activity, you will reflect on interventions and strategies that use a whole population or universal approach. Think of an example of a strategy or intervention in your own country that seeks to address a problem through a universal approach. Which upstream and downstream factors does it address?

Feedback

You might have considered interventions and strategies that include:

• Strategies to reduce smoking. Upstream factors include legislation banning smoking in public places and increasing the cost of smoking. Downstream factors include mass media campaigns on the dangers of smoking and smoking cessation services.
• Strategies to increase the uptake of exercise. Upstream factors include active transport policies, such as walking and cycling, and the provision of new universal affordable sports facilities. Downstream factors include mass media campaigns and community-level intervention seeking to change knowledge, attitudes, and norms to promote exercise.
• Strategies to improve diet. Upstream factors include legislation on health food labelling and regulations on the production of food. Downstream policies include mass media and social marketing campaigns such as the 'Five a Day' campaign used in the UK and other European countries to increase fruit and vegetable intake.
• Sexual health and HIV campaigns. Upstream social and structural factors may include gender inequality targeted through health and empowerment programmes. The mass distribution of condoms and sex education in schools are downstream approaches addressing more 'proximal' risk factors that also exist at a population level.

There are, however, also limitations to a population approach, not least because individual motivation may be reduced by the 'prevention paradox'. Social marketing is one approach that can be used to help sell the benefits of participation to the whole population and avoid public cynicism. Legislation can also change behaviour where individual motivation is limited. Examples of this include legislation to make the wearing of seat belts compulsory in cars and banning smoking in public places. However, there may be ethical issues involved in such legislation. In addition, public perceptions that the state is restricting individual behaviour often makes such legislation unpopular and may make governments reluctant to employ such mandatory behaviour change policies.

Health promotion methods and approaches need to take into account the available evidence on the distribution of risk. In some cases, risk may not be distributed on a normal continuum and/or population approaches could have negative effects on some individuals. The design of interventions also needs to take account of evidence of causality and be aware of the danger of the ecological fallacy. Finally, health promotion interventions need to be designed with the needs of vulnerable groups in mind to ensure that health inequalities are not increased. For example, Frohlich and Potvin (2008) propose that a focus on vulnerable populations should complement a population approach.

Activity 9.3

In this activity, you will consider possible limitations of a whole population or universal approach. Go back to your answer to Activity 9.2. What are the potential limitations of the inventions and strategies you considered? How could they be adjusted to address these limitations?

Feedback

You might have considered limitations and refinements that include:

- Universal strategies to reduce smoking need to take account of the fact that some vulnerable groups are more likely to smoke and less likely to quit than the population as a whole. If smoking rates in the population as a whole reduce at a higher rate than those among vulnerable groups, this will lead to an increase in inequalities in health. Consequently, if this is considered socially or politically undesirable, such strategies need to address the factors that contribute to vulnerable groups smoking, including low income, stress, and isolation.
- Similarly, universal strategies to increase the uptake of exercise need to consider the unequal access of some populations; for example, low-income groups often live in areas that have poorer access to sports facilities and green spaces. Planning and transport policies need to take account of this, for example, by providing safe areas for walking and cycling and bike rental schemes in deprived areas. Sports facilities may need to be subsidized to ensure low-income groups can afford to access them.
- Strategies to encourage healthy eating need to reflect that healthy food choices can be more expensive and that in some deprived areas, there are limited options for buying these healthy foods.
- Sexual health and HIV campaigns may reproduce health inequalities if they do not address underlying problems such as poverty and higher rates of school drop-out among young women from low-income communities. In sub-Saharan African, micro-finance initiatives and conditional cash transfers have been used alongside mass education programmes to address this problem.

Box 9.1 Case study: Teenage pregnancy in the UK

Evidence has shown that teenage pregnancy is associated with adverse social and health outcomes (Ermisch, 2003), even after adjusting for pre-existing social, economic, and health problems (Berrington et al., 2005). As teenage birth rates in the UK were identified as the highest in western Europe (UNICEF, 2007), reducing these rates through an effective teenage pregnancy prevention strategy was identified by the British Government as a priority for 'breaking the cycle' of social exclusion and health problems in low-income communities (Social Exclusion Unit, 1999). National population-level targets for reducing teenage pregnancy were set out in the government's first *Teenage Pregnancy Strategy* launched in 1999 (Social Exclusion Unit, 1999).

In 2006, the UK Department for Education and Schools (DfES) updated the teenage pregnancy strategy. The updated strategy further increased the emphasis on targeted work, identifying 'key risk factors' such as low aspirations and parental background (DfES, 2006). One of the programmes used as part of this targeted approach was the Young People's Development Programme (YPDP). This programme identified young people aged 13–15 years who are deemed by teachers or other care professionals to be 'at risk' of teenage conception, substance misuse, and/or exclusion from school. The programme aimed to reduce teenage pregnancy via an intensive youth work intervention focused on overall 'personal development'. Intervention components included education, training/employment opportunities, life skills, mentoring, volunteering, health education (particularly sexual health and substance misuse), arts, sports, and advice on accessing services (such as family planning). However, targeted interventions may further harm vulnerable young people by labelling them as high risk and/or through iatrogenic social network effects associated with programmes that aggregate them together for long periods of time. When followed-up two years later, those young women in the YPDP programme more commonly reported a teen pregnancy than young women in a comparison group (Wiggins et al., 2009).

In addition, a recent study using UK birth cohort data examined the distribution of risk for teenage motherhood and where in this distribution teenage motherhood outcomes arise (Kneale et al., 2013). As predicted by the Rose hypothesis, key 'risk' factors associated with teenage pregnancy are normally distributed, with targeted approaches therefore likely to be missing the vast majority of 'cases' that the government was aiming to reduce in terms of their population-level targets.

Other studies suggest how whole population approaches (for example, programmes delivered universally through school settings) can be effective for reducing teenage pregnancy and used rather than these targeted approaches. These include interventions to promote teenagers' personal development, self-esteem, and positive aspirations that target whole school populations, such as the US 'learn and serve' programmes which have been found to be effective (Harden et al., 2009). In addition, evidence shows that school ethos interventions and changes to education policy reforms to promote students' engagement at school and expectations for the future can reduce substance use and teenage pregnancy (Bonell et al., 2007). Finally, early years programmes to support parents and foster pre-school children's social and educational development have been shown to have long-term effects on rates of teenage pregnancy (Harden et al., 2009) and could be provided universally.

Summary

The Rose hypothesis proposes the focus of disease prevention should be to reduce the whole population's exposure to key risk factors rather than concentrating on high-risk individuals. This proposal has continued validity for many of the major public health concerns today. The central implication for health promotion is that the Rose hypothesis supports mass interventions, including complex social and structural interventions addressing the upstream determinants of health behaviours. This also raises many questions for health promotion, including: How do we know what is effective at the whole population level? This is a challenge because evidence regarding the distribution of risk is dependent on observational data, which do not provide good evidence about effectiveness. In addition, few people respond to small individual benefits for the greater good of the whole population and there are also political and ethical difficulties in implementing coercive legislation to change behaviour *en masse*. Unless they take account of the specific needs of vulnerable groups, whole population approaches may also contribute to, rather than reduce, health inequalities.

References

Adams, J. and White, M. (2005) When the population approach to prevention puts the health of individuals at risk, *International Journal of Epidemiology*, 34: 40–3.

Berrington, A., Diamond, I., Ingham, R., Stevenson, J., Borgoni, R., Cobos Hernández, M.I. et al. (2005) *Consequences of Teenage Parenthood: Pathways which Minimise the Long Term Negative Impacts of Teenage Childbearing: Final Report*. Southampton: University of Southampton.

Bonell, C. and Fletcher, A. (2008) Addressing the wider determinants of problematic drug use: advantages of whole-population over targeted interventions, *International Journal of Drug Policy*, 19(4): 267–9.

Bonell, C., Fletcher, A. and McCambridge, J. (2007) Improving school ethos may reduce substance misuse and teenage pregnancy, *British Medical Journal*, 334: 614–16.

Charlton, B.G. (1995) A critique of Geoffrey Rose's 'population strategy' for preventive medicine, *Journal of the Royal Society of Medicine*, 68: 607–10.

Davison, C., Davey Smith, G. and Franckel, S. (1991) Lay epidemiology and the prevention paradox: the implications of coronary candidacy for health education, *Sociology of Health and Illness*, 13: 1–19.

Department for Education and Skills (DfES) (2006) *Teenage Pregnancy: Accelerating the Strategy to 2010*. London: DfES.

Ermisch, J. (2003) *Does a 'Teen-Birth' have Longer-term Impacts on the Mother? Suggestive Evidence from the British Household Panel Survey*. Colchester: Institute for Social and Economic Research.

Fletcher, A. (2013) Working towards 'health in all policies' at a national level, *British Medical Journal*, 346: f1096.

Fletcher, A., Gardner, F., McKee, M. and Bonell, C. (2012) The British government's Troubled Families Programme: a flawed response to riots and youth offending, *British Medical Journal*, 344: e3403.

Frohlich, K.L. and Potvin, L. (2008) The inequality paradox: the population approach and vulnerable populations, *Government, Politics and Law*, 98(2): 216–21.

Harden, A., Brunton, G., Fletcher, A. and Oakley, A. (2009) Teenage pregnancy and social disadvantage: a systematic review integrating trials and qualitative studies, *British Medical Journal*, 339: b4254.

Kneale, D., Fletcher, A., Wiggins, R. and Bonell, C. (2013) Distribution and determinants of risk of teenage motherhood in three British cohorts: implications for targeting prevention interventions, *Journal of Epidemiology and Community Health*, 67(1): 48–55.

Lorenc, T., Petticrew, M., Welch, V. and Tugwell, P. (2013) What types of interventions generate inequalities? Evidence from systematic reviews, *Journal of Epidemiology and Community Health*, 67(2): 190–3.

McIntyre, P. and Leask, J. (2008) Improving uptake of MMR vaccine, *British Medical Journal*, 336(7647): 729–30.

Popay, J., Bennett, S., Thomas, C., Williams, G., Gatrell, A. and Bostock, L. (2003) Beyond 'beer, fags, egg and chips'? Exploring lay understandings of social inequalities in health, *Sociology of Health and Illness*, 25: 1–23.

Rose, G. (1981) Strategy of prevention: lessons from cardiovascular disease, *British Medical Journal*, 282: 1847–51.

Rose, G. (1985) Sick individuals and sick populations, *International Journal of Epidemiology*, 14: 32–8.

Social Exclusion Unit (1999) *Teenage Pregnancy Strategy*. London: HMSO.

Stokes, J., Kannel, W.B., Wolf, P.A., D'Agostino, R.B. and Cupples, L.A. (1989) Blood pressure as a risk factor for cardiovascular disease: the Framlingham Study – 30 years of follow-up, *Hypertension*, 13: 113–218.

United Nations Children's Fund (UNICEF) (2007) *Child Poverty in Perspective: An Overview of Child Well-being in Rich Countries*. Innocenti Report Card 7. Florence: UNICEF.

Viner, R., Ozer, E., Denny, S., Marmot, M., Resnick, M., Fatusi, A. et al. (2012) Adolescence and the social determinants of health, *Lancet*, 379: 1641–52.

Wiggins, M., Bonell, C., Sawtell, M., Austerberry, H., Burchett, H., Allen, E. et al. (2009) Health outcomes of youth development programme in England: prospective matched comparison study, *British Medical Journal*, 339: b2534.

Further reading

Hunt, K. and Emslie, C. (2001) Commentary: The prevention paradox in lay epidemiology – Rose revisited, *International Journal of Epidemiology*, 30(3): 442–6.

Rose, G. (1992) *The Strategy of Preventive Medicine*. Oxford: Oxford University Press.

Health communication

Franklin Apfel

Overview

In this chapter, you will learn about how health communication has moved from the margins of public health to being recognized as a core public health operation and competence. Multi-level theoretical and contextual factors driving these changes will be identified. A selection of current health communication practices, approaches, and opportunities, including formative research, framing, social marketing, media advocacy, nudging, health literacy, social media, and m-health will be introduced.

Learning objectives

After reading this chapter, you will be able to:

- understand some of the theoretical and contextual factors that underpin current health communication approaches
- make a case for more investment in health communication capacity
- consider ways to strategically integrate different communication approaches into health promotion, disease prevention and management plans and interventions
- develop a media advocacy plan

Key terms

Communication: Systematic, informed creation, dissemination, and evaluation of messages to affect knowledge, skills, attitudes, beliefs, and behaviours.

Health advocacy: A specific communication strategy that targets decision-makers in health and other sectors and aims to gain political commitment, resources, and support to prioritize and act on health- and well-being-related issues.

Health communication: A multifaceted and multidisciplinary approach to share health-related information with different audiences.

Social marketing: Has been defined as 'the systematic application of marketing concepts and techniques, to achieve specific behavioural goals to improve health and to reduce health inequalities' (French and Blair Stevens, 2006: 2).

What do we mean by health communication?

Health communication has been defined as:

> a multifaceted and multidisciplinary approach to reach different audiences and
> share health-related information with the goal of influencing, engaging, and sup-
> porting individuals, communities, health professionals, special groups, policymak-
> ers and the public to champion, introduce, adopt, or sustain a behavior, practice,
> or policy that will ultimately improve health outcomes.
>
> (Schiavo, 2007: 7)

It is not a one-way communicative act but an iterative social process that unfolds over
time (Obregon and Waisbord, 2012). Health communication encompasses a wide variety of approaches, including: health journalism, blogs, entertainment-education, interpersonal communication, media advocacy, organizational communication, risk and crisis
communication, social communication, marketing and mobilization. It can take many
forms, such as mass multi-media, interactive communications (including mobile telephones and the internet), and traditional and culture-specific communication such as
storytelling, puppet shows, and songs.

Health communication on the margins

While health communication has been identified by WHO and others as an essential
public health operation, it continues to be a neglected subject in health professional
education, poorly resourced in public health agencies and programmes on all levels, and
seen as more of a support function rather than as an integral part of all scientific and
technical work. There are several reasons for this marginal positioning of health communications.

Health communication has often been feared rather than valued. For many health
professionals, ministers, and public health officials, 'no news is good news' because any
news is usually critical and questioning. Officials and agencies are often reluctant to
deal with external communications, distrust journalists, and tend to relegate communications to designated agency public relations/information specialists.

Furthermore, health communication tends to be seen as a softer intervention with
less prestige than more traditional public health activities or clinical treatments. Public
health professionals tend to see vaccines, micronutrients, antibiotics, bed nets, condoms, HIV/AIDS and tuberculosis drugs, and clean water as their tools. They often
assume that if services or 'evidence-based' information are made available, people will
come to use them. Thus the need for communication strategies is ignored. Sometimes
this is correct. However, more often than not, people do not come to use services or
information and the reasons for this are not clear. That is when health communication
people are called in. Health communicators, however, cannot come with ready-made
solutions. Every project requires intelligence gathering and contextual customization.
First (re)actions tend to be more questions than answers. Health communicators' evidence and data are often less clinical and quantitative than those of their medical colleagues and for this reason are seen as 'softer' and less convincing. This leads to lower
prestige of both the professional health communicator and the profession (adapted
from Fox, 2012).

Activity 10.1

This activity encourages you to reflect on some of the challenges of evaluating health communication interventions. Think about how you would go about evaluating a health communication programme. What would be easier to measure? What would be more difficult?

Feedback

It is relatively easy to measure process indicators such as number of newspaper articles published, television 'spots' (public service announcements) aired, billboard posters, pamphlets printed or meetings held. It is also relatively easy to measure reach and determine if television spots are aired or articles are printed in newspapers, blogs or other channels that the intended audience watches, reads or listens to. It is much harder to measure the actual health impact of the health communication programmes. Many health development programmes have short (3–5 year) time spans, which is not long enough for rigorous testing. Confounding factors are often present. Shifts in priorities often work against the ability to carry out longitudinal studies on effectiveness. Few governments or donors are willing to make the levels of investment needed to prove what works in health communication in the same way they would test a new vaccine or a delivery mode for commodities. On top of that, health communication research methodologies are complicated and messy. It is hard to separate control groups and sample groups and not to contaminate one group with another. Adding in ethical considerations makes it even trickier. How can a programme advise one group on a life-saving intervention and not the other in order to test a health communication campaign? How can information be withheld? The short answer is that it can't (Fox, 2012).

While all these difficulties exist, health communication campaigns, particularly those which are integrated into comprehensive control strategies, have been shown to have a significant impact on many key public health challenges, including smoking, alcohol use, use of seat belts, oral rehydration therapy (ORT), support for vaccination programmes, and awareness raising around contraceptives (Wakefield et al., 2010; Fox, 2012).

In addition, health communication does not operate on a level playing field. Health information marketplaces (the real and virtual environments in which people obtain health information) have many actors, agencies, and sources of both information and misinformation. Economic and political interest groups, particularly those that sell hazardous products like tobacco, alcohol, and high-density foods, use their wealth and power to develop and utilize sophisticated targeting and market segmentation techniques to deliver tailored hazard promotion messages to potential customers and those who influence and regulate the markets within which their products are sold. These entities work hard to silence public health communications by framing lifestyle choice issues around rights and individual responsibility, under-emphasizing contextual factors, such as hazard marketing and weak protective health policies, and in some cases trying to directly influence public health agency agendas (Tollison and Wagner, 1993). This is illustrated by the case study on the tobacco industry influencing WHO's communication and action agenda.

Box 10.1 Case study: The tobacco industry's influence of WHO communication and action agenda

Documents from the British American Tobacco Company (Tollison and Wagner, 1993) indicate that they were studying WHO's programme budget in detail and commissioning academics to write articles seemingly in their private capacity that questioned WHO spending priorities. The core of their argument was that WHO 'spending should be concentrated on fighting diseases in third world nations, leaving rich, first world nations to finance their own programs. Hence, WHO funds would go for fighting malaria and cholera, but not go for the campaigns for seat belts or against cigarettes and alcohol'. Concern about documentary evidence pointing to a systematic and global effort by the tobacco industry to undermine tobacco control policy, communication, research and development within the United Nations family, and WHO in particular, resulted in then WHO Director General Dr. Brundtland launching an inquiry into the nature and extent of the undue influence which the tobacco industry has exercised over United Nations organizations such as WHO (Yach and Bettcher, 2000).

Theoretical divides in health communication

Health communication has been informed over the last 50 years by a wide variety of theoretical paradigms used to provide intellectual justification for various interventions. According to Obregon and Waisbord (2012), health communication is characterized by a theoretical divide between information/media effects and participatory/critical theories. The divide is grounded on different conceptions of communication and its place in promoting better health worldwide.

Early health communication theories basically understood communication as the transmission of information and the study of persuasion. Such a view of communication was present in Everett Rogers' (1962) study about the diffusion of innovations. Rogers stressed the significance of people's awareness and knowledge of innovations when they make decisions about whether to adopt them. The media were viewed as agents of positive change, in that they could expose people to 'modern' knowledge and attitudes. Collective behaviours were conceived of as the aggregation of individual practices rather than as distinct phenomena explained by specific dynamics and causes. Such thinking was aligned more with modernistic individualistic biomedical model approaches than the population and system concerns of public health. It took some years for health communication theory to progress towards an amalgam of more public health-oriented constructs that combined informational, participatory, and structural change approaches in complementary ways (Obregon and Waisbord, 2012).

Since then, approaches grounded in social psychological theories have stressed the need to adopt multiple levels of analysis to address the influence of social and policy factors in health behaviours. Chapters 5 and 6 of this book provide further details of these approaches. Examples include the transtheoretical/stages of change model (Prochaska et al., 1994), and the ecological model (Abroms and Maibach, 2008), which propose ways to address a range of individual, social, and policy factors that affect health behaviours and offer a more integrated perspective for analysing a range of social and behavioural determinants, including social networks, social capital, power, participation, and empowerment issues (Obregon and Waisbord, 2012).

Health communication moving to the mainstream

The past two decades have seen rapid changes in national and transnational telecommunication science, technology capacity, and use patterns. The opening of borders, new trade agreements, rapid globalization and urbanization have reshaped health communication marketplaces at all levels. This changing, complex health communication landscape has created unprecedented opportunities and challenges. These include a growing demand for accessible, authoritative, and timely health information.

With increasing education and other social developments in many countries, the issue of health has risen on the political agenda. Increasing access to global news has raised understanding (and sometimes fears) about health-related stories and issues. This has increased expectations and demands, especially during health crises, for rapid access to public health information and advice from policy-makers, national and transnational public health agencies and health services, which is professional, reliable, independent, and transparent.

In addition, the influence of communications on health (and disease) has been enhanced. New transnational media, social marketing approaches, and changes in where and how people seek information have increased opportunities to influence public perceptions, behaviour and choices, and thus the health and well-being of whole populations. Communications, as part of comprehensive public health initiatives, have been credited with reducing some risky forms of behaviour, promoting prevention measures, and influencing healthy choices (UN ECOSOC, 2010; Wakefield et al., 2010; Fox, 2012). A concerted approach to informing about and protecting populations from second-hand smoke has proven successful by undermining former social norms that accepted this risky behaviour. Indoor smoking bans and campaigns push smokers out of social environments, making them feel stigmatized and shunned from mainstream life, literally relegated to the street and to the periphery of their social network so they can continue their habits. These steps have made smoking socially unacceptable and have shown that de-normalizing hazards is possible.

In most countries, however, the aggressive global commercial marketing of tobacco, alcohol, and unhealthy foods continues to lead people towards riskier choices and lifestyles and contributes to the rapidly increasing burden of non-communicable diseases.

Activity 10.2

This activity encourages you to reflect on how health communication is used in practice to counter aggressive marketing of risky products. Make a note of health communication approaches that could be used to counter the aggressive global marketing of risky products and behaviours, particularly those targeting children and youth.

Feedback

Your answer could include a wide variety of innovative approaches to risk factor awareness-raising and behaviour change. These might be initiatives in the workplace, school, health system or community settings. They might involve use of hotlines, new media, mobile telephone technology, interpersonal campaigns, and/or social marketing. Your answer should also acknowledge that communication can also be used to advocate for protective policies and initiatives. Communication initiatives integrated with education and legislative action work best.

The evolution of new media allows citizens and professionals immediate access to relevant and usable information and to contribute and engage. For example, the advent of a global resource such as Wikipedia has demonstrated a completely different model of information provision based on the principles of 'co-creation', where those accessing information actively contribute to its development. This two-way interactive context provides new opportunities for health communication to go beyond simple information provision and harness new technologies to achieve health-enhancing goals.

New behavioural science and ecological approaches have also informed health communication. In recent years, understanding of the factors that influence human behaviour has developed significantly, as discussed in Chapters 5, 6, and 7 of this book. This has highlighted the fact that message communication approaches focused on crafting information and sending messages is not enough to achieve positive impacts on people's choices. New knowledge from across the wider social behavioural sciences, including social marketing, social psychology, behavioural economics, and neuroscience increasingly provides practical, and often cost-effective, solutions to addressing the diversity of behavioural challenges in different populations.

With the growing recognition of the role of health communication has come an increased understanding that inequities in health literacy and information access closely parallel and reinforce the social gradient differentials in disease and mortality patterns in all countries. Poor health literacy, which is more common in lower socio-economic classes, has been shown to lead to less healthy choices, higher risk behaviours, poorer health, higher hospitalization rates, and higher health care costs. The European Health Literacy Project (HLS-EU) showed that nearly every second person (47%) who participated in a survey conducted in eight European countries during 2010 to 2012 had inadequate or problematic health literacy (HLS-EU Consortium, 2012).

These inequities in health literacy have contributed to a growing awareness of the need for stronger advocacy, particularly in the context of financial and economic constraints. Current trends and proposed changes in many countries threaten to reverse progress in public health and widen health inequities within and between countries. Greater communication capacity is needed to support efforts on all levels to ensure that public health values and approaches influence policy debates at all levels.

Current approaches to health communication

Formative research involves testing assumptions through dialogue and conversation with potential users. A crucial step in creating and assessing the potential effectiveness of communication plans and initiatives is to assess baseline knowledge, attitudes, preferences, and behaviours among relevant publics and professionals. This process begins with formative research, a combination of techniques designed to help develop effective messages and choose appropriate channels of delivery and materials.

There are a variety of approaches to formative research, including focus groups, literature reviews, surveys, stakeholder discussions, partnership panels, media audits, in-depth and/or 'intercept' interviews (such as catching people in the hallway), consensus processes (for example, Delphi studies), and the use of internet-based panels of respondents. Small 'focus' groups, for example, selected in such a way as to be representative of groups in society who experience the issue/disease of focus can be convened to elicit feedback about programme planning, provide ideas about strategy, and/or gather reactions to specific messages. Based on feedback from these focus groups, modifications can be made to plans, strategies, and content.

Other uses of formative research include: analysis of target audiences by age, gender or income, known as 'segmentation'; analysis of media habits of the target population so that messages can be placed in the appropriate media channels at an appropriate moment; and an assessment of pre-existing knowledge and attitudes, known as baseline data, so that change can be documented over the time of the interventions. Formative research, when done properly, can reduce some of the uncertainty associated with messages, campaigns, advocacy strategies, and interventions and can enhance the potential methodological validity and reliability and impact of the approaches both for individuals and/or policy-makers and others in the decision stream (Wallack et al., 1993). At the level of population groups, formative research helps ensure an understanding of how different social groups perceive and frame issues and their capacity and resources to act.

Framing/reframing

Framing is 'selecting some aspects of a perceived reality and making them more salient … in such a way as to promote a particular problem definition, causal interpretation, moral evaluation and/or treatment recommendation' (Entman, cited in Chapman, 2004: 362). Framing strategies are at the heart of health communication. The language – both verbal and visual – in which an issue is couched, and the terms in which it is presented, can determine the way in which it is perceived and responded to by both members of the public and policy-makers. This framing creates the context within which all policy debates take place. In a sense, debates over public health policy issues often represent a battle to frame the issue in the eyes of the public and policy-makers in a way most conducive to success for one protagonist or another.

Take, for example, the tobacco and health debate. For many years, the tobacco industry had been very successful in framing public opinion about their product –which kills half of its users prematurely when used as directed – around personal autonomy, choice, and freedom. To achieve this framing the industry hired skilled communication experts to 'spin' public and policy-maker debate around the 'right to smoke' (Chapman, 2007). Within this framing, tobacco smoking ceased to be a health issue and became a matter of personal freedom. In this context, health and social protection concerns fell off the policy agenda. When public health advocates spoke up, they were painted by the tobacco industry as zealots, health fascists, paternalists, and government interventionists (Chapman, 2007; Apfel, 2008/2010).

Key to the success of the WHO's Framework Convention on Tobacco Control (FCTC) was the ability of public health advocates to reframe the issue around public health concerns and shift the attention from public health as interference onto the industry, which had been misleading the broader public for decades as evidenced by their own documents (Glantz et al., 1996). Thus, the slogan 'Tobacco kills. Don't be duped' was used to clearly identify tobacco as a health issue and to shift anger and youth rebellion away from public health interventionists and onto an industry that had for decades intentionally deceived and manipulated people, especially young people, in order to maximize profits.

Communicators blend science, ethics, and politics to frame and reframe, where needed, the dominant understanding and perception of problems. Often this involves shifting perceptions about the cause of ill health outcomes from personal or lifestyle choices, which in essence blame the victim, to focusing on the social policies that shape community behaviours more broadly. In patient safety processes, for example, there has been a framing shift from just focusing on 'blaming and shaming' practitioners who make errors to looking at the system itself, such as how medication is packaged, transported, and labelled, which may have contributed to the error. As such, framing plays a central role in the process of public health policy formation because of the system-level solutions that it implies.

Framing strategies can also be used to gain access and attention for an issue in the media. Here, framing is used to structure stories so they meet the criteria of what constitutes news (for example, relating it to a topical day or event, indicating there is a new breakthrough, controversy, involvement of celebrity, or some other personal angle) and make them more likely to be picked up by news outlets. Structuring a story around these conventions of newsworthiness can enhance the prospects for obtaining media coverage.

Activity 10.3

In this activity, you will explore how framing works in practice for health promotion issues. Vaccination debates are currently framed around safety. This framing appears to reinforce the influence of sceptics and anti-vaccination forces. How might you go about reframing the vaccination debate?

Feedback

There are many possible answers to this question. Building on the discussion of formative research, your answer should include some intelligence gathering aimed at better understanding the perceptions and behaviours of unvaccinated and under-vaccinated populations. This formative research will inform your framing of the issue. Your answer should also acknowledge that different groups might need different messages, framings, messengers or channels of delivery.

Social marketing

Social marketing provides a framework to help integrate marketing principles with socio-psychological theories to develop programmes better able to accomplish behavioural change goals. It takes the planning variables from marketing (product, price, promotion, and place) and reinterprets them for health issues. Box 10.2 provides more detail. A key concept is that it seeks to reduce the psychological, social, economic, and practical distance between consumer and the behaviour. At the core of social marketing is the exchange model, according to which individuals, groups, and organizations receive perceived benefits in exchange for purchased products (for example, condoms, healthier foods) or adopted behaviours (for example, not smoking, safer sex).

Box 10.2 The 'four Ps' of social marketing

Product refers to something the consumer must accept: an item, a behaviour or an idea. In some cases, the product is an item like a condom, and in other cases it is a behaviour such as not drinking and driving. *Price* refers to psychological, social, economic or convenience costs associated with message compliance. For example, the act of not drinking in a group can have psychological costs of anxiety and social costs of loss of status. *Promotion* pertains to how the behaviour is packaged to compensate for costs – what are the benefits of adopting this behaviour and what is the best way to communicate the message promoting it. This could include better health, increased status, higher self-esteem or freedom from inconvenience. Finally, *place* refers to the availability of the product or behaviour. If the intervention is promoting condom use, it is essential that condoms be widely available. Equally important to physical availability, however, is social availability. Condoms are more likely to be used when such use is supported and reinforced by peer groups and the community at large (Wallack et al., 1993: 22).

Social marketers generally believe they address key shortcomings of traditional public health communication campaigns in which target audiences have little input into message development. The major contribution of social marketing approaches has been the strong focus on consumer needs. Consumer orientation means identifying and responding to the needs of the target audience. A primary tool to tailor public communication efforts to specific audiences is formative research (see previous discussion of formative research).

The National Social Marketing Centre in the UK has identified the following six features and concepts as key to a social marketing approach:

1 Customer, consumer or client orientation: A strong customer orientation with importance attached to understanding where the customer is starting from, their knowledge, attitudes, and beliefs, along with the social context in which they live and work.
2 Behaviour and behavioural goals: Clear focus on understanding existing behaviour and key influences on it, alongside developing clear behavioural goals, which can be divided into actionable and measurable steps or stages, phased over time.
3 'Intervention mix' and 'marketing mix': Using a range (or 'mix') of different interventions or methods to achieve a particular behavioural goal. If access related to attending vaccination sessions is identified as a problem, an intervention mix might include changing opening hours, location of services, and SMS reminders to parents.
4 Audience segmentation: Clarity of audience focus using 'audience segmentation' to target effectively. Audiences, for example, can be segmented into subsets based on shared beliefs, attitudes, and behaviours. Interventions are directly tailored to specific (subset) segments rather than relying on 'blanket' or 'spray and pray' approaches. Such segmentation augments traditional targeting using: demographics, socioeconomic and observational data, and epidemiology.
5 'Exchange': Use and application of the 'exchange' concept – understanding what is being expected of 'the customer', the 'real cost to them' (see Box 10.1), and what might be perceived as a valued beneficial outcome of an intervention.

6 'Competition': Use and application of the 'competition' concept – understanding factors that impact on the customer and that compete for their attention and time (NWPHO, 2006).

Box 10.3 Case study: UNICEF and the 2005/2006 avian influenza outbreak in Turkey

During the 2005/2006 avian influenza outbreak in Turkey, UNICEF coordinated a multi-sectoral, multi-agency task force that utilized social marketing techniques to deliver target-specific communications to 'hard-to-reach' high-risk populations. Focus groups and interviews were conducted with mothers living in the rural eastern part of Turkey to understand better their perceptions and risk behaviours (e.g. bringing chickens into the house to keep them warm), to identify messages and incentives that could reduce risk, and media/community channels (e.g. language specific radio and television broadcasts) that could deliver reliable understandable information appropriate to the literacy level of the population. Intelligence gathered also informed advocacy strategies for poultry compensation policies (Apfel, 2006).

Activity 10.4

In this activity, you will practise using a social marketing approach. Breastfeeding has a major role to play in public health, promoting health in both the short and long term for baby and mother. The UK has one of the lowest rates of breastfeeding worldwide, especially among families from disadvantaged groups and particularly among disadvantaged white young women (Dyson et al., 2005: 7). How would you design a social marketing approach to address this challenge?

Feedback

There are many possible approaches to this problem. A social marketing approach would first emphasize taking action to know your 'customers', or target groups, and their knowledge, attitudes, behaviours, and beliefs related to breastfeeding, along with the social context in which they live and work. Target groups could then be appropriately 'segmented'.

A mix of evidence-based interventions would be matched to the audience segment addressed. For example, effective programmes to support behaviour change among low-income mothers would include a combination of peer support, local media campaigns, and targeted community action. To address 'competitive' obstacles related to early cessation of breastfeeding, emphasis should not only be applied to hospital-based interventions to promote higher breastfeeding initiation rates, but to community-based interventions designed to encourage the continuation of breastfeeding to 6–8 weeks and beyond (Dyson et al., 2005).

Media advocacy

Media advocacy involves working with the media to make social changes. In its simplest application, media advocacy asks five key questions (adapted from Wallack et al., 1999):

1 What is the problem?
2. What can be done about it?
3 Who has the authority to do this?
4 Who can influence this authority?
5 What 'mediated' messages will make these influential people act?

The identification of the policy-level authority is key to this approach. This authority is the 'end target' of the media advocacy effort. It is these people with power that communicators/advocates want to influence. They are the primary targets. Media advocates design media campaigns around delivering messages to those people who can influence these primary targets. These influencers are the secondary targets. Advocates want them to act and communicate their messages to the authorities. For example, campaigners concerned about traffic accidents around schools may have identified the school's board of governors as having the power to require traffic-slowing measures to be implemented around the school. They might usefully focus on helping parents, teachers, and students find their voice and deliver messages to those in power. Such action by parents and children may further attract local media and thus serve to influence action by local politicians to introduce traffic restrictions.

In some cases, information alone will be enough to provoke change. In most instances, however, changes will be contested. Media advocates then work with the potential influencers on identifying and strengthening their capacities to deliver more effective messages than their opponents. Delivering messages requires an understanding of how different media channels work and how best to access them.

Common media channels include newspapers, radio, television, billboards, newsletters, web pages, blogs, and email list serves. Each media channel/outlet contains within it several possibilities for coverage. For example, a campaign issue may be covered as a front page story, or in sports, lifestyle, paid advertising, arts, comics, financial, opinion-editorial (known as an op-ed), editorial, special feature or letter to the editor pages of a newspaper. Being aware of all the possibilities is critical to taking full advantage of available resources. Media advocates are above all interested in knowing what channels and outlets their target group of influencers and policy-makers most frequently use.

There are three basic strategies for gaining access to the media: paying for it, earning it, and asking for it. Asking for it usually relates to public service air or print space, often required of media by law as part of licensing requirements. This time and space is free but advocates have little control over when and where their stories will be aired or included. Many are played at less advantageous times, such as the middle of the night, or placed in sections less likely to be read. Nonetheless, this does provide some exposure and it is free!

Paid-for placements are the surest way to see that a message reaches its chosen target. It is the only way to fully control the placement and content of a message, the audience it will reach, and the timing of its dissemination. Canadians for Non-Smokers' Rights used a full-page print advertisement to speak directly to legislators at a critical point in the development of public policy. It included a picture of the then prime minister and his close friend, who had just been appointed President of the Canadian Tobacco Manufacturers Council, beneath a headline that asked, 'How many thousands of Canadians will die from Tobacco Industry Products may be in the hands of these two men.' The advertisement devastated the tobacco lobbying influence by personalizing the issue and making whatever success they could have damaging to the political career of the prime minister. The legislation passed without a problem! (Wallack et al., 1993:89).

Earned, as opposed to paid-for, media coverage, however, is the staple diet of media advocacy. Here the aim is to be proactive to counter the widely held view of health campaigners that when the media calls for a comment, the reporter often already has an angle or 'frame', which may marginalize health concerns in favour of economic and political interests. Proactive strategies require cultivating relationships with members of the local media. Journalists need information and ideas for stories that have importance to the local community. Advocates should think of themselves as resources that can make it easier for journalists to do a good job. Useful accurate data, examples of local activities, a summary of key issues, and names of potential sources can serve this purpose.

Another way to draw news attention is to create it. Opportunities to create news arise every day. The release of a new report or a community demonstration can be turned into engaging news stories. Alternatively, it is possible to 'piggy back' onto the breaking news by finding links with current 'hot' news items and inserting the campaign's perspective. Other coverage includes letters to the editor, op-eds (comment columns that appear near a newspaper's editorial opinion), talk show appearances, and so on. Meetings with editorial boards can be very useful. Shrewd campaigners will be also sensitive to public figures who are espousing important causes. A campaign stands a better chance of publicity if it is supported by a local celebrity (such as a musician, actor or sports person); if that person is committed, they will be willing to take part in events that will attract publicity and could even be the best advocate to encourage journalists to take up the issue. Indeed, a rolling programme of publicity can be achieved by releasing details of new celebrity supporters, whose agents may even encourage them to jump on a popular bandwagon.

Activity 10.5

Design a media advocacy strategy for an institutional or community issue that you feel strongly about.

Feedback

Your answer should go through the five questions above in turn. It should also identify mechanisms, channels, and messengers to deliver the messages you have articulated.

Nudging

'Nudging' is an approach to behaviour change. The term 'nudge' describes 'any aspect of the choice architecture that alters people's behaviour in a predictable way without forbidding any options or significantly changing their economic incentives' (Thaler and Sunstein, 2008: 6).

Marteau et al. (2011) identify a variety of examples of nudging activities:

- Smoking nudges could include making non-smoking more visible though mass media campaigns with the message that the majority do not smoke and most smokers want to stop; and reducing cues for smoking by keeping cigarettes, lighters, and ashtrays out of sight.
- Alcohol nudges could include serving drinks in smaller glasses and making lower alcohol consumption more visible through mass media campaigns with the message that the majority do not drink to excess.
- Diet nudges might include designating sections of supermarket trolleys for fruit and vegetables, and making salad rather than chips the default side-order.
- Physical activity nudges might include making stairs, not lifts, more prominent and attractive in public buildings, and making cycling more visible as a means of transport, for example through city bicycle hire schemes.

Nudging has been criticized by many, however, as either being too paternalistic or incapable of producing sustained change. While it has been suggested as an alternative approach to regulation, some critics believe that 'effective nudging may require legislation, either to implement healthy nudges (such as displaying fruit at checkouts) or to prevent unhealthy nudges from industry (such as food advertising aimed at children)' (Marteau et al., 2011: 228).

Health literacy

Health literacy refers to people's ability to obtain, understand, and use information and is a determinant of their health. In fact, studies show that poor health literacy is a stronger predictor of a person's health than age, income, employment status, education level or race (Weiss et al., 2007: 13). Health literacy is not just determined by an individual's basic literacy skills and motivation. It is also defined by the interaction or alignment of these skills with the demands, complexities, and reliability of information received in the systems within which information is sought. When these systems require knowledge or a language level that is too high for the user, or misinformation is communicated, health will suffer.

Actions and structures within different settings such as health and education systems, media marketplaces, home and community settings, workplaces, and policy-making arenas at all levels, may either facilitate or be a barrier to the development and expression of health literacy skills. Settings and institutions can be more or less health literacy friendly. A wide variety of initiatives are underway in these different settings aimed at differentially enhancing people's health literacy capacities to utilize (navigate through) increasingly complex social and health systems.

Box 10.4 Case study: Local champions

The Liverpool Healthy Cities Project in the UK has initiated a 'local champions' project with the aim of enhancing the capacities of informal community leaders to act as information resources or navigators in areas of high deprivation. These champions, who are active community members, provide interpersonal communication on social services, housing, income support, and health services. More information about the project is available at: http://www.liverpoolpct.nhs.uk/Your_PCT/Decade_of_Health_and_Wellbeing/default.aspx [accessed 19 October 2012].

Social media/Web 2.0

New social media have developed around the increasing public demand for open and interactive communication, sharing and learning, and collaboration. The term Web 2.0 is associated with web applications that facilitate active information-sharing. A Web 2.0 site allows users to interact and collaborate with each other in a social media dialogue as creators of user-generated content. Examples of Web 2.0 include social networking sites, blogs, wikis, and video-sharing sites.

Social media offer new opportunities for the efficient, direct delivery of tailored messages and content to and dialogues with many previously 'hard-to-reach' audiences in a language and format that is adapted to and comprehensible by each audience. Such access has hitherto only been available to highly specialized agencies at great cost. Social media have also demonstrated a capacity to provide important interactive chat and community support opportunities.

Box 10.5 Case study: Patients like me

Patientslikeme.com is an initiative based in the USA that uses a social networking format to enable patients to openly share their data online. This helps to empower patients, who can compare their experiences and make better-informed decisions about the management of their own health. More information about the initiative is available at: http://www.patientslikeme.com/about [accessed 19 October 2012].

Mobile phone health (m-health)

Mobile devices such as mobile telephones, as well as wireless and satellite communications, are giving remote communities an opportunity to be connected and have access to information. Three out of every four people on the planet now have access to mobile telephones and, according to a UN estimate, 64 per cent of all mobile telephone users live in the developing world. The potential for m-health communications is enormous. m-Health is a rapidly evolving communication area and early results support development of it as a powerful, interactive channel for health-related communications. These developments offer exciting opportunities for expanding the availability of health information to underserved populations and countering misinformation rapidly and effectively.

Current uses of m-health communication include citizen science (a variety of activities whereby the public participate in scientific research), education and awareness, disease and epidemic outbreak tracking (providing decision-makers with timely, location-related information), patient diagnostic and treatment support, and health care provider training and communications.

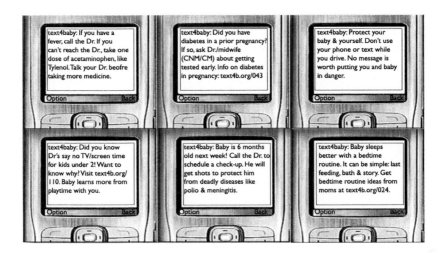

Figure 10.1 text4baby sample messages
Source: Reproduced with permission of text4baby

Box 10.6 Case study: text4baby

The Russian Federation is currently adapting the USA's text4baby initiative that targets high-risk mothers. After texting in their mobile telephone numbers, mothers receive free text messages three times a week that support, inform, advise, and link them to information, support groups in their geographical area (via GPS information), websites, and health and social service facilities. Figure 10.1 shows example messages. More information about the US text4baby initiative is available at: http://www.text4baby.org/ [accessed 19 October 2012].

Summary

This chapter makes the case for the need to strengthen and 'mainstream' communication capacity development as a key public health resource. A variety of approaches using traditional and new media have been described. Just as some soft drinks companies have declared their intention to put a can of cold soda within the reach of every human on the planet, a global community of communication-wise public health practitioners can put reliable and actionable health information within everyone's reach, enhance people's health literacy, make healthier choices easier, and help motivate people to act for health.

References

Abroms, L.C. and Maibach, E.W. (2008) The effectiveness of mass communication to change public behavior, *Annual Review of Public Health*, 29: 219–34.

Apfel, F. (2006) *Making Preparations Count: Lessons from Avian Flu Outbreak in Turkey.* Copenhagen: WHO Regional Office for Europe.

Apfel, F. (2008, updated 2010) *Promoting Health: Advocacy Guide for Health Professionals.* Geneva and Compton Bishop: International Council of Nurses and World Health Communication Associates. Available at: http://www.whcaonline.org/uploads/publications/ICN-NEW-28.3.2010.pdf [accessed 20 March 2013].

Chapman, S. (2004) Advocacy for public health: a primer, *Journal of Epidemiology and Community Health,* 58: 361–5.

Chapman, S. (2007) *Public Health Advocacy and Tobacco Control: Making Smoking History.* Oxford: Blackwell.

Dyson, L., Renfrew, M., McFadden, A., McCormick, F., Herbert, G. and Thomas, J. (2005) *Promotion of Breastfeeding Initiation and Duration: Evidence into Practice Briefing.* London: NICE.

Fox, E. (2012) Rethinking health communication in aid and development, in R. Obregon and S. Waisbord (eds.) *The Handbook of Global Health Communication.* New York: Wiley.

French, J. and Blair Stevens, C. (2006) *Social Marketing Pocket Guide.* London: National Social Marketing Centre for Excellence.

Glantz, S., Slade, J., Bero, L., Hanauer, P. and. Barnes, D. (eds.) (1996) *The Cigarette Papers.* Berkeley, CA: University of California Press.

HLS-EU Consortium (2012) *Final Report Executive Summary (D17), The European Health Literacy Project.* Maastricht: Maastricht University. Available at: http://www.fgoe.org/projektfoerderung/gefoerderte-projekte/FgoeProject_1412/52050.pdf [accessed 18 January 2013].

Marteau, T.M., Ogilvie, D., Roland, M., Suhrcke, M. and Kelly, M.P. (2011) Judging nudging: can nudging improve population health?, *British Medical Journal,* 342: d228.

NorthWest Public Health Observatory (NWPHO) (2006) *Synthesis: Bringing Together Policy Evidence and Intelligence.* Liverpool: NWPHO. Available at: http://www.nwph.net/nwpho/publications/Synthesis_6_Socialmarketing.pdf) [accessed 15 January 2013].

Obregon, R. and Waisbord, S. (eds.) (2012) *The Handbook of Global Health Communication.* New York: Wiley.

Prochaska, J.O., Norcross, J. and DiClemente, C.C. (1994) *Changing for Good: The Revolutionary Program that Explains the Six Stages of Change and Teaches You How to Free Yourself from Bad Habits.* New York: William Morrow.

Rogers, E.M. (1962) *Diffusion of Innovations.* New York: Free Press.

Schiavo, R. (2007) *Health Communication: From Theory to Practice.* San Francisco, CA: Jossey-Bass.

Thaler, R.H. and Sunstein, C. (2008) *Nudge: Improving Decisions about Health, Wealth, and Happiness.* New Haven, CT: Yale University Press.

Tollison, R. and Wagner, R. (1993) *World Health and the World Health Organization.* BATCo Document June 23, 1993:500899074 (cited in Yach and Bettcher, 2000).

United Nations Economic and Social Council (ECOSOC) (2010) Health Literacy and the Millennium Development Goals. United Nations Economic and Social Council (ECOSOC) Regional Meeting Background Paper (abstracted), *Journal of Health Communication,* 15(1): 211–23.

Wakefield, M., Loken, B. and Hornik, R. (2010) Use of mass media campaigns to change health behaviour, *Lancet,* 376(9748): 1261–71.

Wallack, L., Dorfman, L., Jernigan, D. and Themba, M. (1993) *Media Advocacy and Public Health: Power for Prevention.* Newbury Park, CA: Sage.

Wallack, L., Woodruff, K., Dorfman, L. and Diaz, I. (1999) *News for a Change: An Advocate's Guide to Working with the Media.* Newbury Park, CA: Sage.

Weiss, B.D., American Medical Association and AMA Foundation (2007) *Health Literacy and Patient Safety: Help Patients Understand.* Chicago, IL: AMA Foundation.

Yach, D. and Bettcher, D. (2000) Globalisation of tobacco industry influence and new global responses, *Tobacco Control,* 9: 206–16.

Further reading

Social Marketing Institute: http://www.social-marketing.org/success/cs-floridatruth.html [accessed 10 August 2011].

World Health Organization Regional Office for Europe (2012) *European Action Plan for Strengthening Public Health Capacities and Services*. Copenhagen: WHO.

Further information on the tobacco industry can be found at the Legacy Tobacco Documents Library (LTDL), which enables researchers to search, view, and download more than 13 million documents created by the tobacco industry concerning scientific research, manufacturing, marketing, advertising, and sales of cigarettes at: http://www.library.ucsf.edu/tobacco [accessed 25 March 2013].

Glossary

Beneficence: Doing good; active kindness.

Communication: Systematic, informed creation, dissemination, and evaluation of messages to affect knowledge, skills, attitudes, beliefs, and behaviours.

Community capacity building: Enabling people in communities to participate in actions based on community interests.

Community health competence: The degree to which a community is health-enabling and responsive.

Community response: The combination of actions and steps taken by community members for the public good, including the provision of goods and services.

Conscientization: The development of a critical consciousness, a better understanding of the inequalities that exist in the world, particularly in relation to self.

Determinants of health: The range of factors that combine together to affect the health of individuals.

Disciplinary power: A modern and more concealed form of power that works through systems of knowledge and practice, which, by creating standards of 'normality' and 'abnormality', induces people to constantly examine and adjust themselves and others according to such norms.

Discourse: Bodies of language, knowledge, and practice that constitute the very things they appear to describe.

Eugenics: The science of human heredity, informed by evolutionary theory. In the early twentieth century, eugenics was concerned with racial improvement and the prevention of degeneration.

Evidence: The available body of facts or information indicating whether a belief or proposition is true or valid.

Evidence-based medicine: The conscientious, explicit, and judicious use of current best evidence in making decisions about the care of individual patients.

Evidence-based public health: The conscientious, explicit, and judicious use of current best evidence in making decisions about the care of communities and populations in the domain of health protection, disease prevention, health maintenance and improvement.

Health advocacy: A specific communication strategy that targets decision-makers in health and other sectors and aims to gain political commitment, resources, and support to prioritize and act on health- and well-being-related issues.

Health behaviour: Actions undertaken by an individual that have an effect (positive or negative) on health.

Health communication: A multifaceted and multidisciplinary approach to share health-related information with different audiences.

Health promotion: The process of enabling people to increase control over, and to improve, their health (Ottawa Charter for Health Promotion, 1986).

Iatrogenic effect: An unintentional harmful effect of an intervention or policy.

Inequalities in health: Differences in health status between different populations and social groups.

Inequities in health: A term that can be used to describe inequalities in health that are deemed preventable.

Liberalism: The rights of the individual should be respected to enable society on a whole to benefit from the full potential of all its citizens.

Neo-liberalism: A modern variation on liberalism, typically used in the context of the role of the state, emphasizing market-based solutions to problems rather than public intervention.

New public health: Form of public health that developed from the 1970s onwards. It emphasized risk, prevention, and individual behaviour as a cause of disease.

Non-maleficence: A principle based on avoiding the causation of harm.

Normative: Behaviours and practices that are viewed as 'normal' or 'correct' in a particular social context.

Participatory learning and action: An approach for learning about and engaging with communities using participatory and visual methods to facilitate a process of collective learning and action.

Phenomenology: A qualitative research paradigm, derived from the writings of philosophers such as Husserl and Buber, that focuses on the lived and subjective experience of phenomena. It seeks to describe and appreciate how people themselves understand and give meaning to their own experiences.

Plato's Republic: An ideal society governed by those best qualified to do so.

Policy: A course or principle of action adopted or proposed by an organization or individual.

Policy agenda: The list of subjects or problems to which government officials and those close to them are paying serious attention to.

Prevention paradox: The paradoxical situation whereby a preventative measure that significantly benefits the whole population offers little to each individual.

Primary health care: Health services and care delivered at the local level often through community health workers, which has been particularly important in the global south from the 1970s onwards.

Rose hypothesis: Proposition of Geoffrey Rose that because risk is normally distributed on a continuum, prevention strategies focusing on the whole population are likely to be more effective that those focused on high-risk groups and individuals.

Salutogenesis: An approach focusing on factors that support human health and well-being, rather than on factors that cause disease.

Self-efficacy: Belief in one's ability and capacity to achieve a goal.

Semiotics: The study of signs and symbols that aims to deconstruct their coded meanings. Includes signs and symbols in any medium or sensory modality (e.g. words, images, sounds, gestures, and objects).

Social capital: The social benefits that derive from social networks and collaboration between people, and their shared values and norms of behaviour.

Social constructionism: A critical conceptual framework that understands things that are generally thought to be exclusively natural as being socially produced.

Social determinants of health: The social, economic, and environmental factors that impact on health behaviours and determine the health status of individuals or populations.

Social epidemiology: The field of epidemiology that examines the social and spatial distribution of health outcomes and the social determinants of health outcomes.

Social inequities: Differences in opportunity for different population sub-groups.

Social marketing: The systematic application of marketing approaches to achieve specific voluntary behavioural goals.

Social medicine: Form of public health developed in the inter-war years. Concerned with the effect of social conditions on health and mortality.

Social norms: Pattern of behaviour in a particular group, community or culture, accepted as normal and to which an individual is expected to conform.

Socio-economic status: An individual's place in the social hierarchy according to their level of income, education, occupation, and/or where they live.

Targeted approach: A health promotion strategy or intervention targeted at individuals or groups who are identified as being at higher than average risk of disease, injury or other adverse health outcomes.

Theory: Systematically organized knowledge devised to analyse, predict or explain observable phenomena that could be used as the basis for action.

Utilitarianism: A theory of the good (whatever yields the greatest utility or value) and a theory of the right (the right act is that which yields the greatest net utility).

Whole population approach: A health promotion strategy or intervention aimed at the whole population in question, rather than targeted at specific high-risk individuals or groups. Also sometimes known as a 'universal' or 'population-level' approach.

Index

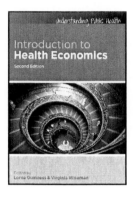

**GEORGESON & PAYLER
INTRODUCTION TO HEALTH
ECONOMICS**

Second Edition

Lorna Guinness and Virginia Wiseman

9780335243563 (Paperback)
September 2011

eBook also available

This practical text offers the ideal introduction to the economic techniques used in public health and is accessible enough for those who have no or limited knowledge of economics. Written in a user-friendly manner, the book covers key economic principles, such as supply and demand, healthcare markets, healthcare finance and economic evaluation.

Key features:

- Extensive use of global examples from low, middle and high income countries, real case studies and exercises to facilitate the understanding of economic concepts
- A greater emphasis on the practical application of economic theories and concepts to the formulation of health policy
- New chapters on macroeconomics, globalizatio**n and health and provider payments**

www.openup.co.uk

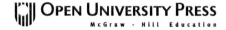 **OPEN UNIVERSITY PRESS**
McGraw - Hill Education

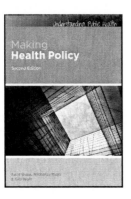

MAKING HEALTH POLICY
Second Edition

Kent Buse, Nicholas Mays and Gill Walt

9780335246342 (Paperback)
2012

eBook also available

Part of the Understanding Public Health series, this bestselling book is the leading text in the field. It focuses on how health policy is made nationally and globally, clearly explaining the key concepts from political science with a wide array of engaging examples.

This edition is fully updated to reflect new research and ways of thinking about the health policy process. Written by leading experts, this clear and accessible book addresses the "how" of health policy making in a range of international settings.

Key features:

- International perspectives
- Clear explanation of complex ideas/concepts
- Updated with latest policy developments and relevant changes to procedure

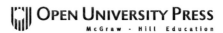
www.openup.co.uk — OPEN UNIVERSITY PRESS — McGraw · Hill Education